A Blessing In Disguise
The Lizard
The Secret Of Spiritual Growth

Forward

This book was created to help people survive Pandemics. This book has plenty of information on how to avoid getting sick. It also has information on how to cope with it mentally. It even provides guidance on how to deal with the crisis spiritually. This book is designed to help people cope with the physical , mental and spiritual crisis that comes with the effects of pandemics and how people have have had to change their lifestyle.

This book is written for families. The writings within it are meant to be shared by both adults and children. There is even a fantastic story for the very smallest of children (Adaboo and The Greatest Love of All). One of the main chapters centers on families (Chapter 2 The Power of Family). There is also another chapter on The Power of Working as a member of A Community. There is another chapter on The Power of Learning Life Lessons in Times of Crisis.

We have gathered a collection of writings that will provide readers with an opportunity to learn and grow during the crisis. It will both entertain you and provide guidance on protecting you physically, give you nourishment for your spirit, and food for thought. The pandemic that created the need for this volume may be with us for only a few months or maybe several months. Many of the writings contained in this volume will stand the test of time and serve to sustain you in any other crisis that happen in your life.

The Physical, Mental and Spiritual Pandemic Survival Guide
A Family Oriented Survival Guide

By Mark Wilkins, The Prophet of Life & Dr. Goose.

Table of Contents:

Chapter 3 The Power of Acting as a Member of the Community

Chapter 4 The Power of Life Lessons in Times of Crisis

We hope that you thoroughly enjoy reading this book. It was a pleasure for us to create it. It is our greatest hope that you and those you love not only survive pandemics but thrive and grow during your time of isolation.

Sincerely,
The Staff and Authors
at Loveforce International Publishing Company

Chapter 1 The Power of Basic Knowledge

How to Keep A Level Head in Times of Crisis

Life presents us with many crisis. Some are personal. Some are regional. Some are national. Some are global. A rampant pandemic usually begans as a local crisis. Then it grows to a national crisis. Then it becomes a global crisis. As a pandemic progresses, the hospitals overflow and the deaths mount we must remember that this crisis too shall pass.

One pandemic is not worse than others that have come in the past. They may seem to be to many of us but in reality there are many others that were far worse. Every pandemic however has the capacity to become more widely spread than those of the past because of the ease and affordability of travel. There are some who may use a pandemic as an excuse for some nations to become isolated but isolation is nothing more than withdrawal from the humanity. It is a denial of your culture, your heritage and your identity from the human race. Cultures that isolate fail to contribute to humanity and their stories become lost to the ages. Their stories die with them.

We live is a world of interdependency whether you like it or not. You can either admit the fact and begin to look at the world and humanities problems from a global perspective or deny it at your own expense. What harms one society harms every society. What began in China is now all over the world. Don't blame the source of a pandemic. Blame the rest of the world. The rest of the world doesn't often much care about an epidemic when it is confined to one area or even one nation. Then, befor eyou know it, it's everywhere. Suddenly the rest of the world cares.

Some will use a pandemic as a gripe session. Others see it as an opportunity. It can be an opportunity to grow. It can be an opportunity to learn what it has to teach us. Often, Pandemics will force people to self-isolate. The amount of time they have to isolate is difficult for some. They are away from their work, their friends and some family members. Yet they are with some family members. They have a lot more freedom. Not to go places physically but to go places mentally and spiritually.

Self-isolation is the time to watch, listen, and read things you haven't had time to before. It is the time to build relationships with those you live with. It is the time to be thankful for all that you have instead of resentful for all that you don't. It is the time to do these things because now you have time. You may not get an opportunity again for some time, so use it wisely.

So, how do you keep a level head in times of crisis? Take it one day at a time. Do what you can and don't worry about what you can't. Be thankful for what you have been given instead of resentful for what you have not. Know that this too shall pass and that better things are on their way. Cherish those near and dear to you and if you lose them in this time of crisis know that they knew you loved them and cared about them. There is no gift more powerful than to leave this world knowing that you were loved and that people cared about you. Nothing except the gift of life.

What is a Pandemic?

Most dictionaries define it as an outbreak of a disease over a whole nation or over the entire world. Any disease can become a pandemic. It is also possible for diseases to jump species (go from animals to people or from people to animals. This is because as the human population explodes and human expansion into wilderness areas increases people live in closer proximity to wild animals and that proximety can cause a disease jump between species.

Groups at Higher Risk for Severe Illness

In most pandemics there are certain groups that are at higher risk for getting a severe form of whatever disease has become a pandemic. those who have a high-risk for severe illness are often the elderly (65 and older) and people who have pre-exiting conditions which weaken their immune system. Like asthma, a serious heart condition, HIV/Aids, cancer, people with kidney and liver problems, people who are severely obese, people who have diabetes, people who are steroid users and heavy smokers.

Things You can do to Protect Your Family During A Pandemic

The best thing you can do is stay home. Go out only to buy things essential for your survival. Minimize your number of trips out, and the length of time you are out when you are on them. When you enter a public place, talk as little as possible and move as quickly as possible. Touch as little as possible. Stay at least 6 feet away from everyone. Wear face mask and gloves. Gloves can help protect you from physically touching something with the virus on it but not if you touch your face, nose, eyes or mouth while you are wearing the gloves. When you don't have gloves use an alcohol-based hand sanitizer after every time you touch something.

Wash your hands with soap and hot water for at least a 20 second lather vigorously rubbing your hands and fingers together every time you touch something that others may have touched. Wash your hands every time you come inside the house from anywhere outside of the house. If soap and water aren't available, use a hand sanitizer that contains at least 60% alcohol. Pour it over every surface of your hands and fingers and rub your hands and fingers together vigorously until they are dry.

Keep shoes used outside near front entrance to your home. Spray down with disinfectant before you put them in the house. As soon as you enter (in your stocking feet) remove your pants, shirt & jacket put in laundry basket then go to the bathroom, wash your hands thoroughly, then take a hot shower with soap and water.

Inside the house clean and disinfect surfaces frequently touched. Clean and disinfect surfaces like phones, remotes, tables, doorknobs, light switches, countertops, handles, desks, keyboards, toilets, faucets, and sinks daily. Follow the instructions on the product label. Spray or pour spray products onto a cleaning cloth or paper towel instead of spraying the product directly onto the cleaning surface (if the product label allows).

Avoid sharing personal household items such as cups, towels brushes and tooth brushes. Walk around in pajamas and socks or slippers. Only wear inside clothing inside the house not things you have worn outside until they are thoroughly washed. If someone in your home is sick, have them stay away from the rest of the household to reduce the risk of spreading the virus in your home. Cancel your travel, especially if it is cruise travel. Have a staycation instead of a vacation.

Coughing & Sneezing Etiquette

When you are at your home and / or whenever you are not wearing a face mask you should cough or sneeze into a facial tissue or if one is not available, the inside of your elbow especially if you are wearing a long sleeve shirt. If you use a facial tissue be sure and throw it in the trash immediately. Then wash your hands thoroughly with soap and hot water or, if that is unavailable, use hand sanitizer that has at least 60% alcohol.

Chapter 2 The Power of Family

It's Only Love

Love
It's only love
Just a simple emotion
Yet to some it's everything

It can make you feel like somebody
When nobody knows your name
It takes the stormy part of your existence
And soothes you until it's tame

Love
It's only love
Just a simple emotion
Yet to some it's everything

It fills your world with joy
Gives you a warm feeling inside
It gives your life meaning and purpose
It makes you mellow and satisfied

Love
It's only love
Just a simple emotion
Yet to some it's everything

Fatherhood

Every, June 21st it's Father's Day in America. Having spent time in America, I will take this day to write about fatherhood. My father left my mother after their divorce. My sister and I spent many years growing up in foster homes. I had no real father figure to look up to. I gravitated towards men who had qualities I admired so I could observe them and learn what manhood was about. A neighbor taught me how to tie a tie. A teacher taught me the importance of written expression. A boss taught me the importance of courtesy and developing a work ethic. All of these temporary surrogate fathers made an impact on me.

Then one day, I realized that there had always been one father figure present in my life all along. God. I know now that God is neither male nor female but when I was young, I needed a father figure, so for these purposes, God was a male. I thought about the kindness God bestows upon all beings. I worked on developing my innate kindness. I thought about how God works to right wrongs and I endeavored to use my writing ability as a tool to help right the wrongs in this world. I thought about how God loves all living beings and developed a sense of love for all things, people, animals, plants and even bugs.

I have known many men in my life. Some have abandoned their children. Others are excellent fathers. I try and influence those who have abandoned their children into get back into their children's lives in any way they are able. I frequently praise the fathers who are excellent fathers. I really admire them. I applaud them. While they believe that they are doing a wonderful thing for their family, they are also doing a wonderful thing for humanity. Through parenting, they are shaping the future of humanity by developing great people who will contribute to humanity. Above all, they are doing God's work.

Fathers are special people. Any man can be a sperm donor. It takes a great man to take the time, effort and devotion to be a father. To all the great fathers out there you are appreciated. Enjoy your day.

I'll Be Your Rock

When you need me I'll be there
You'll never have to ask
You'll know I care
When your star dreams come crashing down on your head
I'll put them back where they belong
Or create better ones instead
CHORUS
I'll be your rock
The one person you can lean on
And always depend on
When others talk
I'll be your rock

When the world turns its back
I will stand by your side
 Even when the deck is stacked
When you are lost and far away from happiness
I'll be your beacon through the storm
A helping hand in your distress
CHORUS
I'll be your rock
The one person you can lean on
And always depend on
When others talk
I'll be your rock

Plan Your Household Defense Against A Pandemic

You have been drafted whether or not you like it. A Pandemic has declared war on humanity and all of us must prepare to defend ourselves and those we love against it if we are to survive. As a family, you can plan and make decisions now that will protect you and your family during a pandemic.

The first thing you can do is stay informed. Stay informed by getting up to date information about the Pandemic both internationally, nationally and in your local area. Make a list of organizations in your area including local organizations that can help you with healthcare and support services. You can also put together a list of people you may need to contact in case of an emergency including first responders (police, fire, ambulance) teachers, employers and local public health officials. Call ahead for any appointments you have (including medical appointments) to see if they are still keeping appointments and if so, under what circumstances.

Part of staying informed is keeping track. Keep track of local events, the hours businesses that are essential for survival (banks, places that sell food, gas, medicine) are open. Many businesses have closed or have different hours they are open. Many have rules like limiting the number of people who can be there at one time. Keep track of all those things..

The next thing you can do is prepare for possible sickness. The first way you can prepare for possible sickness is to stock up on essentials like toilet paper, water, cleaning and disinfectant supplies, bleach, alcohol, chlorine wipes and hand sanitizer that is at least 60% alcohol based. If people or pets in your household require medication stock up on that medication as well. If you have pets don't forget to stock up on pet food as well. If you have children stock up on things for them to do indoors.

The second way you can prepare for possible sickness is to identify people in your household who are at the greatest risk for severe illness and provide them extra protection. Identify a room in your home as a quarantine room for whomever gets sick. Try and stay at least 6 feet away from them even when you are providing care for them, if possible. Wear gloves when you are providing care for them.

The third way you can prepare for possible sickness is to create and maintain health conscious habits. Get in the habit of keeping up a prevention routine for everyday living, for when you have to leave and go outside of your home and for when you come back from outside. Get in the habit of cleaning and disinfecting surfaces regularly and of avoiding touching your nose, eyes, and mouth. Get in the habit of washing your hands the proper way frequently.

As you are engaging in your cleaning protocols, you may, at times find that you run out of cleaning & disinfecting supplies. Here is something that you can do in an emergency if you have either bleach or alcohol that is at least 70%.

Making a solution with your household bleach:
To make a bleach solution, mix:

- 5 tablespoons (1/3rd cup) bleach per gallon of water

OR

- 4 teaspoons bleach per quart of water

Always follow manufacturer's instructions for application and proper ventilation. Check to ensure the product is not past its expiration date. Household bleach that has not expired will be effective against coronaviruses when properly diluted. Never mix household bleach with ammonia or any other cleanser.

Alcohol that is at least 70% will work as an adequate disinfectant.
Ensure solution has at least 70% alcohol.

The fourth way you can prepare for possible sickness is find out what the awrning signs and symptoms are for the pandemic from a reliable source like the Centers for Disease Control (CDC) or the World Health Organization (WHO). Once you know what they are, then watch for the warning signs. If anyone in your household has them, quarantine them in your quarantine room. Do not allow them to leave your home unless they are going for medical care. Get in touch and stay in touch with your doctor in case more severe signs develop. Call to ensure that you have the correct hours medical care, including nearby hospitals are open and what alternative hospitals or medical care is available when the nearby doctor / hospital is closed.

If you or a member of your family develop emergency warning signs for a severe form of a pandemic disease, get medical attention immediately. Always avoid taking an infected person by public transportation (taxis, buses, rideshare companies) as they are likely to spread the disease. Always call ahead to let the medical office or hospital you are visiting know that the person you are bringing possibly has the pandemic disease so they can prepare for them. This helps insure that the disease doesn't spread to the medical staff and other patients.

Send a Smile

Children building dreams
In the sand
Lovers strolling
And holding hands
Old people lie beneath a tree
half asleep
Sentimental memories
Are theirs to keep

Teens singing to the rhythm
Of a beat up guitar
Reaching out to be somebody
But proud of what they are
Their parents sit watching
Under sunny skies
Hoping tomorrow's promises
Will be realized

If you see life with an open heart
And open mind
You'll find we're all the same inside
There's so much we can share
Send a smile
Show you care

The Terror

He saw the Terror when he first entered the department store. The Terror was with his weary, single mother and frightened younger brothers. At just four years old, the terror wanted desperately to get his way. His mother dreaded taking him anywhere but none of her relatives would watch him and she didn't dare leave him alone with a babysitter. The Terror was yelling and kicking at the shopping cart while his mother and brothers stood looking at him, powerless to do anything about his rage.

"You better give me the toy I want!" He demanded. "You better give it to me or you'll be sorry!" He continued.

The man went about his shopping and didn't give the terror a second thought. He walked over to the checkout lines when he finished a half an hour later. He was dismayed to find that there was a long line at each of the six cash registers. The exit door was about 50 feet to the right of the sixth cash register. He decided to get in line at the first register, the farthest from the exit door because that line was about two people shorter than all the other lines. Within seconds, he heard a familiar sound.

"Get me my toy! Get it!"

He looked over to where the noise was coming from and two registers over, close to the front of the line he saw The Terror yelling. His beleaguered mother tried to calm him down. Many of the people in the checkout lines were looking at The Terror and the commotion he was making.

"It's okay sweetie, we'll get you a toy next time." She said calmly.

This bit of news angered The Terror.

"Next time?" He questioned. "No! I want it NOW!!"

The Terror began whining and crying and kicking the shopping cart furiously in a tantrum.

"Why can't I have the toy? Why? I want it NOW!!!!" He screamed at a pitch so high some of the people in the lines had to put their hands over their ears.

With that particular scream, literally everyone in all of the checkout lines began looking at The Terror and his mother.

"Now dear, we don't have enough money to get you a toy this time." She said in a calm voice.

The Terror's eyes seemed to enlarge. He began screaming.

"I hate you! I HATE YOU! You are the worst mommy in the whole world! I'm never going to forgive you! I'll hate you for this forever! Do you hear me? Forever!!!!" He screamed as he tantrumed and cried simultaneously.

This went on for the five minutes that the mother and her children waited in line to pay for their things. During the course of the five minutes, people waiting in not only her checkout line, but all of the checkout lines began staring at them with angry disgust. Some of them began muttering to themselves and others began talking about it. They said things like:

"Why doesn't she just smack that brat?"

"Doesn't she have any consideration for others?"

"Why does she even take that kid in public?"

"She should have left that brat a t home."

"Why doesn't she just leave her crap in the cart and leave the store?"

Then the mother got up to the register. She paid for her things as the cashier loaded them into her shopping cart. Just as she was about to roll out of the store, The Terror laid down in the middle of the floor. She told him to get up but he refused. He began kicking and screaming.

"I'm not going anywhere until I get my toy! You can't make me go. You are a bad mommy! BAD MOMMY!!!!" He yelled between kicks.

It was three long minutes of listening to the tantrum before the man got up to the cash register. In those minutes, people who checked out voiced their disapproval to the mother as they left. The poor mother turned red with embarrassment. Seeing his mother turn red emboldened The Terror, who in turn, kicked and screamed even louder while lying on the floor.

"Stay here and do that all you want, I am still not buying that toy for you!" She yelled back at him.

In response, The Terror began weeping loudly and uncontrollably.

Having paid for his things, the man began walking towards the exit. Instead of shuffling past The Terror as everyone else did, he stopped next to him and began to talk to the boy's mother.

"May I talk to your son?" He asked.

"Why do you want to talk to him?" She replied.

"I think I might be able to calm him down." He said.

"You're not going to hit him are you?" She asked.

"No." He replied.

"Or yell at him?" She asked.

"No, I'm just going to talk to him calmly, as you do." He replied.

"Good luck with that." She said. "Sometimes he stays like this for a couple of hours." She added.

"What's the boy's name?" The man asked.

"Bobby." His mother replied.

The man walked over to the boy so that he was towering directly above him. Then he calmly called the boy's name.

"Bobby." He said.

The boy ignored him. The boy's mother gave the man a look that if translated into words, would have said "I told you so." Undeterred, the man looked down at the boy.

"Is that you Bobby?" He a bit louder said in a calm tone of voice.

The boy looked up at the man.

"Do I know you?" He asked the man.

"I live down the street from you Bobby and I always thought you were a very smart boy!" The man stated.

"I am smart." Bobby replied confidently.

"Oh, I agree with you Bobby, really I do, but you see all of these people Bobby?" He said as he pointed towards the people in the checkout lines.

Bobby looked up at all of the people in the checkout lines. He saw the anger and scowls of disapproval on their faces. "Those people?" Asked Bobby.

"Yes those people." The man replied. "Well, they all think that you are not smart at all." The man continued.

"Why?" Asked Bobby.

"Well, you have been screaming and crying and carrying on for a long time now, and, do you have the toy you want Bobby?" The man asked.

"No." Replied Bobby.

"It seems to me Bobby that a smart boy would see that this isn't working for him and try something different. Are you a smart boy Bobby?" The man said.

"I am smart!" Bobby stated emphatically with a whine in his voice.

"Then Bobby…" The man said. "Why don't you try something different?"

"Like what?" Asked Bobby.

"First, let's get up off of the floor, shall we? I'll help you up." The man said as he extended his hand to Bobby. Bobby grabbed onto the man's hand. The man lifted Bobby up as easily as a child can lift a feather. Once Bobby was up on his feet, he looked at the man.

"Now what?" Asked Bobby.

"First, you must earn the respect of all the people who are looking at you." The man said.

"How do I do that?" Bobby asked.

"By telling them you are sorry for not acting like the smart boy that you really are." He said.

"I can't do that!" Bobby replied.

"Sure you can Bobby and when you do, you can see how your words magically affect all of them." The man said.

"Magic?" Bobby asked.

"Yes Bobby, because words have power. The words you said before had the power to make all of these people upset with you but saying you are sorry will have the power to change the looks on their faces." The man said instructionally.

Bobby looked at all of the people in the checkout lines.

"I'm sorry." He said.

The looks on everyone's faces changed from anger to forgiveness.

'Wow!!!" Exclaimed Bobby with shocked joy. Then he looked at the man again.

"Now what?" Bobby asked again.

"Now you must say you are sorry to your mommy and brothers so you can see the magic work on them too." The man said.

"I'm sorry mommy, you really are a good mommy." Bobby said.

Then he hugged his two brothers while saying "Sorry guys."

As Bobby apologized to his siblings, his mother looked up at the man and mouthed "He's never apologized to me before." The man turned to leave. He began to walk towards the store exit. Bobby, sensing that the man was leaving, called out to him.

"Hey mister!" Bobby shouted.

The man turned around.

"What about my toy?" He asked. "How do I get it?" He continued.

The man walked back over to Bobby.

"When was the last time you acted like you did earlier and actually got a toy?" He asked.

"I think I was two." Bobby replied after pausing to think about the question.

'So now, if you want to get a toy, try being a good boy and doing everything your mommy tells you to do and maybe you will get a toy *sometimes*." The man said.

"Sometimes?" Asked Bobby with a hint of anger in his voice.

"Yes." Said the man. "But sometimes is less time to wait than two years is. You will get what you want more often by being a good boy, at least that's what a smart boy would do and aren't you a smart boy Bobby?"

"I am a smart boy." Bobby replied happily.

Keep the Home Fires Burning

Feels like a million miles though I know it ain't
Being without you
I might as well be serving time

I'd like to hold you close to me
But it's going to have to wait
My job keeps taking me further on down the line

But keep the home fires burning
Burning on for me
When you're lonely know you're not the only one

Keep the home fires burning
And know that I will be
Heading home just as soon as my work is done

Gee, I'm glad I caught you in
It's great to hear your voice
How have you been? Say, tell me all the news

I'd really like to get away
But I don't have any choice
I swear that I will find a way to make it up to you

Keep the home fires burning

Touch

It's getting hard for me to express the things I feel
There's so much that my heart would like to say
I would really like to get closer to you
I'd like to send some special thoughts your way

Touch
Keep in touch
It means so much
Cause I really care about you
Touch
I need to feel your touch
You mean so much
And it's rough being without you

What I wouldn't give to have you hear with me right now
To gaze into your eyes once again
To hold you in my arms deep into the night
To feel the warm smoothness of your skin

Touch
Keep in touch
It means so much
Cause I really care about you
Touch
I need to feel your touch
You mean so much
And it's rough being without you

What to do if a family member becomes infected.

Here are some things to do to help ensure that other people in your home remain disease free. Make sure the isolated individual(s) are in a quarantine room. Make sure they wear a face mask whenever they are exposed to other people including in your house. Try and stay at least 6 feet away from them even when you enter the quarantine room to provide care for them. Wear gloves whenever you enter the quarantine room or are providing service for them.

Keep Things clean and disinfected. Frequently clean all surfaces that are touched often, like counters, tabletops, and doorknobs. Use household cleaning sprays or wipes according to the label instructions. Wash laundry thoroughly. If laundry is soiled, wear disposable gloves and keep the soiled items away from your body while laundering. Wash your hands immediately after removing gloves.

Protect non-infected people. Keep the infected individual(s) isolated. Avoid having any unnecessary visitors. Don't allow the infected individual(s) to leave your home and / or go out in public.

Provide symptom treatment for the infected individual(s). Make sure they drink a lot of fluids to stay hydrated and get plenty of rest at home. Over-the-counter medicines may help with symptoms (check with your doctor).

What to do When Quarantine Ends

Everyone feels differently after coming out of quarantine. There are different types of feelings your loved ones may be experiencing. They may feel mixed emotions, including relief after quarantine. They may experience Fear and worry about their own health and the health of loved ones. They may have some lingering stress from the experience of being stuck in quarantine dependent upon others. They may feel sadness, anger, or frustration because friends or loved ones had fears of contracting the disease from contact with them. They may feel guilty about not being able to perform normal work or other duties during quarantine.

Children may also feel upset or have other strong emotions if they, or someone they know, has been released from quarantine. These may cause stress. Let them know it wasn't their fault that they got the disease. Reassure them that the quarantine was to protect others in the household and did not diminish everyone's love and affection for them. Let them know that the person who was in quarantine is now ready to rejoin the group and participate as they normally would.

A Smart Spouse

Bryan and Annie had been married about four years. Bryan was fifteen years older than 27 year-old Annie. Annie and Bryan had a big dog. Annie had the habit of allowing the dog to climb up on her lap, touch his nose to hers and give her a big lick on her face. Bryan never really minded it. It was just one of those peculiar things a spouse does that the other spouse put up with and learns to ignore.

Annie's mother was visiting for a week. She worked very hard making a turkey dinner. The three of them sat down at the table and began eating. Suddenly, their dog Sparky put his front paws on Annie's lap and hoisted himself up. She turned her face towards him and he touched his nose to hers. Then he give her face a great big lick. The dog lowered himself down and laid down besides Annie.

Annie's mother was horrified by what she had just witnessed.

"What a pig!" she yelled. "What a pig you are Annie!"

Then she looked at Bryan. "What do you think boychic? Which of them is a pig, your dog or my daughter?"

Bryan thought for a moment before he responded.

"If you're asking me which one is a pig, my wife or my dog, the pig is always my dog." He said.

Annie chuckled with glee. "What a wonderful husband I have!"

Annie's mother quipped "But Annie is intelligent she has a brain and should know better. The dog is just a dumb dog?"

"Because tonight, when I go to sleep," Bryan replied, "I want to sleep in my bed with my beautiful, loving wife instead of in the doghouse with Sparky."

Muscle Man

A husband and wife had been married for many years. The husband had long since passed his prime and rarely exercised. He still liked to think of himself as a handsome, well-built man. One day, his wife touched his belly, which had expanded several inches over the years, and said "Flabby".

The man took this statement to heart and resolved to do some-thing about it. He detested exercise. The next time he saw her hand move towards him he tensed his muscles. She didn't say he was flabby. Over time, the man developed the habit of tensing up whenever his wife's hand moved towards his body.

One day the wife decided to test her husband. She moved her hand towards his shoulder, he tensed up. It was rock hard. She moved her hand towards his arm. He tensed up there too, she giggled. She moved her hand to the small of his back, he tensed up there too. She giggled again. Her hand gently roamed toward the back of his thigh. He tensed up there too. She laughed.

Then, with a twinkle in his eye, he said "How do you like your muscle man?"

"I wish the man I was feeling was the man I was married to." She replied with a smirk.

Coping with Stress

Pandemics can be stressful for people. Fear and anxiety about a disease can be overwhelming and cause strong emotions in adults and children. Coping with stress will make you, the people you care about, and your community stronger.

Everyone reacts differently to stressful situations. How you respond to the outbreak can depend on your background, the things that make you different from other people, and the community you live in.

People who may respond more strongly to the stress of a crisis include older people and people with chronic diseases who are at higher risk for a severe form of illness from a pandemic, children, people who have mental health conditions and people who have problems with substance abuse. People who are helping with the crisis response to the pandemic, like doctors and other health care providers, and first responders also accumulate stress.

There are many different signs of stress during a pandemic. Here are a few examples. People under stress can show fear and worry about their own health and the health of their loved ones. They can have changes in sleep or eating patterns. They can have difficulty sleeping or concentrating. You might see increased use of alcohol, tobacco, or other drugs. Any of these things individually or any combination of them can lead to worse health and / or a worsening of chronic health problems they already have.

The Emergency Phone Numbers for Every Nation in the World

If you, or someone you care about, are feeling overwhelmed with emotions like sadness, depression, or anxiety, or feel like you want to harm yourself or others call an emergency help line. A global list of Emergency help lines for Medical Emergencies and / or ambulance for every nation is listed below:

911 in the U.S., Saudi Arabia, Ethiopia, Kenya, Liberia, Uganda, Tristan da Cunha, Iraq, Jordan, Fiji, Gum, The Marshall Islands, Micronesia, palau, Tonga, Tuvalu, Belize, Costa Rica, Panama, Argentina, Bolivia, Ecuador, Paraguay, El Salvador, Honduras, The Bahamas, Cayman Island, Grenada, Navassa Island, St. Kitts & Nevis, St. Lucia, St. Vincent & The Grenadines, US Virgin Islands, Barbados, Bonaire, The Dominican Republic, Armenia, American Samoa, Bermuda, Canada, Mexico, Peru, Uruguay, Philippines,

112 in India, Angola, Benin, Burundi, Burkina Faso, Cameroon, Ghana, Guinea-Bissau, Mayotte, Nigeria, Reunion, Sao Tome & Principe, Afghanistan, Bhutan, East Timor, Kazakhstan, Kuwait, Tajikistan, Turkmenistan, Aland Islands, Belgium, Bulgaria, Cyprus, Denmark, Estonia, Faroe Islands, Finland, Germany, Georgia, Gibraltar, Greenland, Guernsey, Iceland, Ireland, Isle of Man, Jersey, Italy, Latvia, Lithuania, Luxembourg, Malta, Moldova, Netherlands, Northern Cyprus, Portugal, Romania, Slovenia, Spain, Turkey, French Polynesia, New Caledonia, Vanuatu, Clipperton Island, Guadeloupe, Martinique, Saint Pierre & Miquelon, Falkland Islands, French Guiana,

999 in the UK and Singapore. Ascension Island, St. Helena, Seychelles, Somalia, Sudan, South Sudan, Zambia, Zimbabwe, Akotiri and Dhekelia, Bahrain, Bangladesh, Myanmar, Hong Kong, Macau, Malaysia, Qatar, UAR, Kiribati, Samoa, Guyana, South Georgia & Sandwich Islands.

000 Australia, Cocos Island, Christmas Island,

15 France, Mali, Morocco, Niger, Monaco,

18 Guinea, Senegal,

101 Israel, Mauritania, Uzbekistan,

102 Nepal, Maldives,

103 Russia, Belarus, Azerbaijan, Ukraine, Transnistria, Abkhazia,

104 Serbia, Hungary,

110 Syria, Sri Lanka,

111 New Zealand, Papua New Guinea, Nauru,

114 Tanzania, Mauritius, Eretria,

115 Iran, Suriname, Viet Nam, Pakistan, Equatorial Guinea,

116 Haiti, Gambia,

119 Indonesia, Japan, Republic of Korea, Democratic People's Republic of Korea, Cambodia, Sri Lanka,

123 Colombia, Egypt, Madagascar,

124 Bosnia and Herzegovina, Montenegro,

128 Nicaragua, Guatemala,

144 Austria, Liechtenstein,

155 Slovakia, Czech Republic

194 Croatia, Kosovo, Republic of North Macedonia,

195 Honduras, Laos,

912 Rwanda, Curacao,

Nations with their own unique emergency number:

120 People's Republic of China, 14, Algeria, 19 Djibouti, 102 Nepal, 104 Cuba, 105 Mongolia, 110 Jamaica, 113 Norway, 116 Andorra, , 117 Mozambique, 118 San Marino, 121 Lesotho, 127 Albania, 130 Cape Verde, 131 Chile, 132 El Salvador, 140 Lebanon, 144 Switzerland, 150 Western Sahara, , 166 Greece, 185 Ivory Coast, 191 Yemen, 192 Brazil, 198 Tunisia, 811 Trinidad and Tobago, 977 Swaziland, 991 Brunei, 997 Botswana, 998 Cook Islands, 1220 Central African Republic, 1300 Gabon, 1515 Libya, 1669 Thailand, 8200 Togo, 9999 Oman, 10 177 South Africa, 772-03-73 Comoros, Chad 2251-4242

Here are a couple of other things to remember while coping with stress. People with preexisting mental health conditions should continue with their treatment and be aware of new or worsening symptoms. Taking care of yourself, your friends, and your family can help you cope with stress. Helping others cope with their stress can also make your community stronger.

Things You can do to Lower The Level of Stress In Your Home

There are several things you can do to lower stress levels in your home. Take breaks from watching, reading, or listening to news stories, and social media that are reporting on the current Pandemic. Hearing about the pandemic repeatedly can be upsetting. Take care of your body. Take deep breaths, stretch. Try to eat healthy, well-balanced meals, exercise regularly, get plenty of sleep, and avoid alcohol & drugs. Make time to unwind.

Try to do some other activities you enjoy. Connect with others by phone and through social media. Learn something new. You can study it on the internet. Learning something new will take your mind off of isolation and make time pass by more quickly.

If you are feeling isolated or depressed talk with people you trust. Talk to them about your concerns and how you are feeling. Call your healthcare provider if stress gets in the way of your daily activities formore than a day or two.

Sharing the facts about a Pandemic and understanding the actual risk to yourself and people you care about can make an outbreak less stressful. Sharing accurate information about the pandemic you can help make people feel less stressed. When people are less stressed they are more likely to connect with you.

A Tribute to Mothers Everywhere

No Matter what language you speak

Mother Is spelled LOVE

Where would you be without your mother?

You would not be here.

In many cultures mothers are seen as the child bearers

But in reality they are the Life Givers

Because they not only bear children but nurture and raise

them as well

And for many, a mother's love is the only human love that

is unconditional

And the only love from another human being that has

endured throughout their lives

Even those who don't know who their father is know who

their mother is

So if your mother is alive

Hug her

If she is far away, call her

You know she would always do the same for you

If she has passed on

Remember her

Say a prayer for her

She may not have been perfect

But she always did the best she could

I will close with lyrics about mothers

From a song I wrote Called "Hope Is The Answer"

Woman is a mother

She's got a lot of mouths to feed

Feels like a martyr

Frustration is what she bleeds

So many disappointments

Yet her faith it keeps her strong

Kids need someone to look up to

In times of desperation

To all the mothers out there………….. :)

The Best Gift to Give a Child

What is the best gift to give a child?

It's not something you have to spend a lot of money on.

It's not something you have to spend a lot of money on.

It is something you will have to spend time on.

The best gift to give a child is the gift of high positive self-esteem.

Girls with high positive self-esteem are less likely to sleep around and become pregnant in their teen years.

Boys who have high positive self-esteem are less likely to become victims of bullying.

Kids who have high positive self-esteem are less likely to succumb to peer pressure become drug addicted or gang members

And are more likely to believe in themselves and not afraid to think out of the box or act independently.

All of these things are benchmarks of success in school, in work and in life.

Positive High Self-esteem can be built by:

Praising the good things your child does.

Encouraging your child to try new things.

Supporting the things you child wants to try and to do.

Showing your child unconditional love no matter what they have done.

So save your money.

Take the time

Make the effort.

Give your child positive high self-esteem.

Adaboo and The Greatest Love Of All

Adaboo was a prince in a great kingdom. He, however, was a lesser known prince. For, while all of his brothers and sisters were known for doing big and important things, Adaboo was little and the only thing he was known for was being cute.

One Morning, Adaboo woke up with a question on his mind. The question was: What is the greatest love of all? Adaboo decided that he would spend the day trying to find the answer to this question.

Adaboo left his bedroom and went to his mother. He spoke to her.

"Mama, what is the greatest love of all?" he asked

'There is no greater love than the love a mother has for her child. When you are in pain, she comforts you. When you need someone to talk to, she listens. Even when the whole world is against you, she is always for you. She only wants the best for you. A mother's love is the greatest love of all because it never ends." She replied.

Adaboo thought that was a wonderful answer to his question. He wondered, however, would others agree?

Adaboo walked out into the courtyard and towards the palace gates. As he approached the gate, a soldier guarding the gate spoke to him.

"And where are you off to little prince?" He asked.

"I am in search of the answer to a question." Adaboo Replied.

"What question is that?" The Soldier Asked.

"What is the greatest love of all?" Adaboo Replied.

"Why that question is easy to answer!" Exclaimed the soldier.

"It is?" Questioned Adaboo.

"Why sure, it's the love of your Nation!" The Soldier Exclaimed proudly. "Soldiers like myself love our nation so much, we are pledged to defend it. We would even give our lives for it." He added.

"That is a wonderful answer!" Adaboo Replied. "But I think I will go out into the city and see if everyone else agrees with you." He Added.

The soldier let Adaboo pass and he walked into the city.

After a few blocks, Adaboo came upon a lawyer on his way to court. Adaboo motioned for the lawyer to stop and the lawyer did just that.

"Sir, What is the greatest love of all?" Adaboo asked.

"It must be the love for the law. For in the law, there is justice. In Justice there is fairness. In fairness, there is happiness because everyone wants to live in a world where things are fair." The Lawyer replied.

Adaboo thanked the lawyer, told him that he gave a legally wonderful answer to his question and kept on walking. After a few blocks, he came upon a library. He climbed up two flights of stairs and went in through the back entrance. He soon saw an interesting woman. She was hidden behind stacks of books. As Adaboo drew closer he could see that many of them were open and the woman was reading intensely. He guessed that she was a scholar. Adaboo walked over to her and asked her his question.

"Excuse me madam." He said. "What is the greatest love of all?" He concluded.

The woman put aside the book she was engaged in reading and pondered for a few moments before speaking.

"The greatest love of all is the love of knowledge, for in knowledge is the answer to all questions including yours." She replied. Then she thought again for a moment. "So, I would have to say that the greatest love of all is the love of knowledge." She concluded.

Adaboo told the woman that she indeed had a scholarly wonderful answer to his question. He thanked her, decided to depart from the front library and began walking down the front stairwell. Just across the street from the library was a market square. On the landing about half way down the stairwell, there was a landing which overlooked the market square. A man with an easel, a canvas, paints and a brush was at the landing. He was painting a picture of the market square. Adaboo decided to ask him his question. Adaboo stopped at the landing and began speaking. "Sir". He began. "What is the greatest love of all?" He continued.

The artist stopped his work for a moment and while gazing at the market square, he answered Adaboo. "The love of beauty is the greatest love of all." He Replied. "Without beauty, without art or music or poetry, the world would be a very ugly and boring place." He continued.

Adaboo thanked the man, told him his answer was simply wonderful and continued on his journey. He crossed the street and entered the market square. While walking through the market square, he came upon a very old man sweeping the street. He decided to ask him the question too.

"Sir." Adaboo began. "What is the greatest love of all?" He concluded.

The old man stopped sweeping. He leaned on his broom and gazed off into the distance at something that must have been very far away because Adaboo didn't see anything extraordinary nearby.

"I…Would….have to say…." He began slowly. "It would be the love of your work." He continued.

"The love of your work?" Asked Adaboo.

"Yes, because you spend most of your life working and if you don't love your work, you will have a miserable life." He said. Then he continued. "When you look at me, what do you see?" He asked Adaboo.

"I see a man who sweeps the street." Adaboo Replied.

"That is what most people see, a man who cleans up after others." He Replied. "I have been sweeping this street for 60 years. Street sweeping is the only job I know. It is the only job I have ever known. I see it as an important job because if no one cleaned the street, the street would be filthy. Filthy streets attract insects and rats. Insects and rats bring disease. They don't bring disease to this street because I am here to sweep it and keep it clean. I love my job. I believe it is an important job. So I live a happy life, knowing that my job is important. Most people look at me and just see a street sweeper but I know I am a super hero." He continued.

"A Superhero?" Adaboo asked.

"Yes, I am a guardian of the public health and because I love my work and I am happy in my work I would say that the greatest love of all is the love of your work." He concluded.

Adaboo thanked the man, told him that he had an absolutely wonderful answer to the question and continued walking through and beyond the market square thinking about the new things he learned about street sweepers being superheroes.

After a few more blocks, Adaboo came upon a hospital. As he walked up the street towards the hospital he saw a doctor getting out of her car. Adaboo walked up to her. "Excuse me doctor." He said. "Can I ask you a question." He continued.

"What a cute little boy!" She exclaimed. "Are you sick?" She asked.

"No Madam." Adaboo Replied. "I just want to know the answer to a question, the question is: What is the greatest love of all?"" He Concluded.

The Doctor answered without hesitation.

"I would have to say it is the love of humanity. As a doctor I heal the sick. I make people better. I have dedicated my life to others and to making them well again."

Adaboo told her she had a selflessly wonderful answer. He thanked her and then turned and walked back towards the palace, for it was late afternoon and he wanted to be home before night fell. After a few blocks he passed a school. A teacher was watching his students get onto a school bus to take them home. Adaboo stopped next to the teacher.

"Excuse me teacher." He said. "What is the greatest love of all?" He asked.

The teacher replied immediately.

"The greatest love of all is the love of teaching because teachers build the future one child at a time." He Replied.

Adaboo told the teacher he had a wonderful answer and continued on his way back to the palace. After a few blocks, he saw a young couple walking hand in hand. He stopped them and asked them the question.

"Excuse me, what is the greatest love of all?' He Asked. Without hesitation they both answered together.

"The greatest love of all is the love of your spouse." They Replied.

"Your spouse will always protect and support you." Said the man.

"Your spouse will always honor and respect you, love and cherish you, as long as you have your spouse you will feel loved." Said the Woman.

"And when you feel loved…" Said the man. "That's the greatest love of all."

Adaboo told the couple that they have a lovingly wonderful answer. He thanked them and continued up the street. After walking a while, Adaboo came upon a Holy Man.

"Excuse me." Adaboo Said. "I have been walking all day long asking a question and I would like to ask you." He Continued.

"Go ahead," Said the Holy Man. "Ask it and I will answer it if I can." He concluded.

"What is the greatest love of all?" Adaboo asked.

The Holy Man reflected for a moment. Then he replied. "The greatest love of all is the God's love, for God created heaven and earth. It is God's will that allows us to be born and sustains us each day. God's love surpasses all other loves combined and therefore, God's love is the greatest love of all."

Adaboo told the Holy Man that he had a reverently wonderful answer. He thanked him and continued on for the sun was setting and the palace was in sight.

Several minutes later, Adaboo walked back through the palace gates. He was too tired to eat, so he just went to his bedroom. He took a hot shower and put on his pajamas. As his mother kissed his forehead and tucked him in for the night,   Adaboo realized that he didn't get one particularly perfect answer to his question. He did, however, get many wonderful answers.

Adaboo realized that the greatest love of all was different for each person. He found it interesting that everyone he asked knew what the greatest love of all was for them. This meant that everyone knows love and everyone has love. For Adaboo, the greatest love of all was drifting off to sleep knowing that the world is so full of love.

Bobby

Bobby, hero of the water bag wars

The most fantastic

Tree house explorer

Bobby, director of the soap box plays

Captain of the puddle pirates

On rainy days

Most folks call her a tomboy

But I know that will change in time

When she sheds her jeans for a prom dress

Adulthood isn't far behind

Bobby, winner of the three legged race

In King of the Hill

No one can take her place

Bobby, leads the sandlot sluggers in home runs

But she's the last one home for dinner

When the day is done

Ways You can Relieve Stress in Children

If you are a parent or a caregiver for children, keep in mind that children often base their reactions to stressful situations on how they see the adults around them reacting. Parents and caregivers can provide the best support for their children by dealing with a pandemic calmly and confidently. Parents can be more reassuring to others around them, especially children, if they are knowledgeable and prepared.

While not all children respond to stress in the same way, there are some common changes to watch for younger children. Excessive crying or irritation, is one thing. Returning to behaviors from their early childhood (for example, toileting accidents or bedwetting) is another.

Teenage children may experience changes that are common to them. One is poor school performance or avoiding school work. Another is difficulty with attention and concentration. A third sign is avoiding of activities they enjoyed in the past. A fourth is use of alcohol, tobacco, or other drugs.

There are also some changes that are common for all children, no matter what their age. One is excessive worry or sadness. Another is developing unhealthy eating or sleeping habits. A third is irritability and "acting out" behaviors. A Fourth is unexplained headaches or body pain.

There are many things you can do to support your children and relieve their stress. First, reassure your children that they are safe. Let them know it is okay if they feel upset. One way to help them feel normal is to keep up with regular routines. If schools are closed, create a schedule for learning activities and relaxing or fun activities. Stay connected with family members who don't live with you. Let your children know how you deal with your own stress so that they can learn how to cope from you. Finally, you can model the behaviors you want your children to have by taking breaks, getting plenty of sleep, exercising, eating well and remaining calm.

Children can sometimes misinterpret what they hear and can be frightened about something they do not understand. You can take time to talk with them about the pandemic. Be sure to answer questions about the current pandemic with facts, in a way that your children can understand. There are things you can do to help your minimize your children's stress level in regards to over exposure to pandemic coverage or exposure to websites not meant for children. One is limiting your family's exposure to news coverage of the event. Using your child's computer settings to regulate what they can see, hear and do on social media. It's okay to communicate with friends, for example, it's not okay to go to websites with gory pictures of people who have died during the pandemic. These suggestions can help stop children may misinterpreting what they hear. They can help stop children from being can be frightened.

I Couldn't Love You More

Do you realize
The miracle that you are?
You are the brightest shining star
In the special universe
Within my heart

Have you ever noticed
The magic you love contains?
It banishes all pain
And makes your world beautiful
Again

In the deepest regions of my soul
I am sure
 Yes, I know
I couldn't love you more

Do you realize
How gifted you must be?
So full of energy
Your imagination turns
Into reality

Have you ever noticed
The sunshine you create?
You positively motivate
And cause all of life
To celebrate

In the deepest regions of my soul
I am sure
 Yes, I know
I couldn't love you more

Hold Onto Love

People will play with your emotions
Time will put you through changes
It's only when you let them get to you
That these things in life become dangerous

Stay in touch with your feelings
No matter what others do or say cherish the love that lives
in your spirit
Don't let anything wear it away

Hold on to love
Even if it's the only thing you've got
Hold onto love
Don't you ever give it up

Pressure can work to break down your heart
Frustration can tear at your soul
That's when you've got to fight even harder
Not to grow callas and cold

Stay in touch with your feelings
No matter what others do or say cherish the love that lives
in your spirit
Don't let anything wear it away
Hold onto love

I Just Want To Be Good To You

VERSE 1
I don't want to own you
Don't want to control you
Oh I, yes I, want to be good to you
I don't want to make you sad
And I'll never treat you bad
I want to be good to you
Real love is not possessive
It doesn't know of jealousy
I gladly gives without thought of taking
Just like the love between you and me

I just want to be good to you
Good to you
I just want to be good to you
For good

VERSE 2
I don't want to hold you back
I want you to face the fact
That I just want to be good to you
And when hard times visit you
I'll comfort and see you through
Cause I just want to be good to you
True love is something that sustains you
It makes you glad to be alive
It helps you realize your hopes and your dreams
Together, side by side

I just want to be good to you
Good to you

I just want to be good to you
For good

Chapter 3 The Power of Acting as a Member of the Community

A Matter of Perspective

Three old men were sitting on a bus bench. To pass the time they had a conversation comparing how hard their childhoods were. While the first two old men were talking, the third just sat listening.

The first old man said "When I a kid, I had to walk three miles to school every morning."

The second old man said "I had to walk four miles."

The first old man said "There were no traffic signals, I risked my life crossing the street."

The second old man said: "You had streets? I had dirt roads. I risked my life with every step I took because a car could run me over at any time."

The first old man, who was by now upset said: "I had to walk in sub-zero, freezing temperatures!"

The second old man said "I did too and our weather was so cold, my jacket froze!"

The first old man, figuring out how the second old man bested him, chimed in: "You had Jackets!"

The second old man replied: "Yes we had jackets but we were so poor my jacket was made out of paper bags."

The first old man, in an obviously lame attempt to best the second one, shouted: "Yeah? Well, when I was a kid I walked to school in temperatures so cold my shoes froze!"

To which the second old man replied: "You had shoes?"

The Third old man, who had been sitting quietly during the entire conversation suddenly spoke; "You had feet?"

Then he opened his jacket and revealed two legs cut off at the knee caps.

Sometimes we look at life from the perspectives of our own problems and in so doing, ignore how fortunate we really are.

Plain Speaking

VERSE 1
Let's take the CON out of conversation
Let's put the HUMAN back into humanity
Let's put the yoU back in communication
And the PERSON back in personality

Plain speaking
Saying exactly what we mean
Plain speaking
Not hiding our words behind a screen

VERSE 2
Let's take the NO out of innovation
Let's take the MOCk out of democracy
Let's put the Pay back into occupation
And the RESPONSE back in responsibility
Plain speaking

VERSE 3
Let's put the VISION back into television
The FACT back into satisfaction
The CANDID back into candidate
And the ACT back into action
Plain Speaking

Plain speaking
Saying exactly what we mean
Plain speaking
Not hiding our words behind a screen

I'm Beyond Your Perception Of Me

VERSE 1
It's just the tip of the iceberg you know
You've only scratched the surface
What stands before you is an infinite soul
A life that's filled with purpose
I'm more than
You'll ever know
More than you see

CHORUS
I'm beyond
Your perception
Of me

VERSE 2
You've known me for the longest time
I live and work beside you
You've discounted this heart of mine
Even though it beats true
My love is brighter
Than the stars
Deeper than the sea

CHORUS
I'm beyond
Your perception
Of me

VERSE 3
We walk alone, along the path

Find kindred souls in passing
Learn lessons in the aftermath
Of scars that are everlasting
Life is journey
Of becoming
All we can be
CHORUS
I'm beyond
Your perception
Of me

Reducing Stigma Reduces Tension

Often during pandemics there is a tendency towards blaming. Blaming can pit one group of people against other groups. This increases tension. It is important to remember that people who are from but do not live in a place that has reported cases during a pandemic are not at greater risk of spreading it than other people in your nation. People who have not recently been in an area of an ongoing spread of the disease, are not at greater risk of spreading it than other people in your nation. People who have not been in contact with a person who is a confirmed or suspected case of the pandemic are not at greater risk of spreading it than other people in your nation. Blaming and stigmatizing these people does not protect you from the pandemic it only subjects others to prejudice.

Public health emergencies, such as a pandemic are stressful times for people and communities. Fear and anxiety about a disease can lead to social stigma towards people, places, or things. Stigma and discrimination can occur when people associate a disease with a population or nationality, even though not everyone in that population or from that region is at risk for the disease. Stigma can also occur after a person has been released from quarantine even though they are not considered a risk for spreading the pandemic to others.

Stigma raises tension, creates stress and hurts everyone by creating fear or anger towards other people. Some signs of stigma include social avoidance or rejection, denial of healthcare, education, housing or employment, public condemnation and even physical violence. Stigma affects the emotional and mental health of stigmatized groups and the communities they live in. Stopping stigma is important to making communities and community members stronger and more able to fight the current pandemic. Everyone can help stop stigma related to it by knowing the facts and sharing them with others in your community and by speaking out when you see stigma occurring.

There are other ways you can help stop stigma and help strengthen your community. You can raise awareness about the pandemic without increasing fear by sharing accurate information (from the CDC & / or WHO) about how the pandemic spreads. Speak out against negative behaviors, including negative statements on social media about groups of people, or the mistreatment of people who pose no risk from regular activities. Be cautious about the images that you share with others. Make sure they do not reinforce negative stereotypes.

The Throwaway Mentality

We live in a world that has a throw away mentality. Things are made to be thrown away. Packaging for common household products (toothpaste, laundry detergent, canned foods), are made to be thrown away. Large products like furniture, building supplies and consumer electronics are also destined for generally short lifespan followed by a trip to the trash bin.

This throw away mentality, whether it was created by corporations with planned obsolescence, advertisers creating the desire to have the new and improved version or consumers driven by peer pressure to keep up with our friends and neighbors, this throw away mentality has been woven into the fabric of our global culture. Unfortunately, it extends beyond mere products and into human relations.

What may have started out as a desire to make things bigger and better has evolved into an overall approach to life in general? People are now looking beyond products and looking at relationships with others living beings as throw away as well.

People are throwing away their pets. They get a pet, the pet doesn't conform to what they expected and they give it to the pound, throw it out of the house or drive it to another town or the middle of nowhere and let it go. In the past week friends have told me about two families, one who were going on vacation and didn't want to spend money to board their seven year old dog, so they brought it to the dog pound. The other family dropped their eleven year old dog off at the vet to be euthanized on their way to Disneyland. The left it up to the Vet staff to help the poor animal overcome the feeling of abandonment as they gave it a lethal injection, while they enjoyed a ride on the Pirates of The Caribbean.

People are also throwing away their relationships with other people. Friendships end just when the friend is in need. Romantic relationships end when one partner discovers a flaw in the other or because the two parties are arguing. Marriages end because people don't have the time or desire to work on their relationship. In some nations 50% of all marriages end in divorce. When there are children involved, some parents abandon the relationship with their children out of anger or trepidation at dealing with their former partner.

The thing that most people don't think about when they are practicing a throw away mentality is that thrown away doesn't mean problem solved. Thrown away means the problem is taken from the sight of the one doing the throwing and left for someone else to take care of. The items we throw away go to landfills. Pollute the ocean or just hang around until they are, little by little disintegrated over a period of years. The relationships we throw away produce traumatized animals and broken people. Until we as individuals and humanity as a race begin to change our way of thinking we will continue to throw away things, animals and people until we become something less than human. Next time you are throwing away something, be it a product, a pet or a relationship with another person, think about where the throw away will really end up and how much pain it will cause the human family.

Different

If I march to the beat of a different drum
What's wrong with that?
And if I disagree with where you're coming from
Don't get upset

It takes all kinds of people to make the human race
And everyone fits in their own way

There's no right
No wrong
There's just different
Culturally speaking

A lot of the bickering in this world
Could be stopped tonight
If we just begin to respect
Each other's way of life

It takes all kinds of people to make the human race
And everyone fits in their own way

There's no right
No wrong
There's just different
Culturally speaking

One World One People

VERSE 1
Things are rough all over these days my friend
Sometimes it seems hard times will never end
But when realities nightmares come creeping
At times when I'm not sleeping
I call on inner strength to make them pass away
Cause I know,
Yes I know
In my heart of hearts I know
That everything will be okay

Cause we've got one world
One people
Two sexes
Both equal
sixteen billion eyes
Eight billion souls see through them
But just one race
And that is human

People looking to find the solutions to
Problems that confront them both old and new
In times of desperation
Inner communication
Brings forth an understanding light
And they'll know
Yes they'll know

In their heart of hearts they will know
That everything will be alright

Cause we've got one world
One people
Two sexes
Both equal
sixteen billion eyes
Eight billion souls see through them
But just one race
And that is human

How Everything is Connected

One day, while I was watering my backyard, The Lord taught me the following lesson. As I was watering the grass, I noticed part of the tree root popping out above the grass about 20 feet from the tree. It was then that The Lord came to me and said:

"If you wish to water the tree you must not only water it at the base of the tree but you should also water where it's roots crop up all over the yard." Said The Lord. "Stop and look." He continued, "at all of the places where the tree root crops up in your yard."

I did so. I found about a dozen places.

"If you don't water all of those places", The Lord continued "The tree will wither and die in the places where you do not water. Not watering the entire tree, in all of the places where its root crops up hurts the tree. In this way, the tree is connected to your yard and your yard to the tree." The Lord pointed out.

"This tree in your yard can also represent the tree of life on this planet." The Lord continued, "All life on this planet is connected. If you neglect one part of the life on this planet, be it an individual or an entire species of plant or animal, you harm all life on this planet because all of life on this planet is connected just as the roots of this tree are connected."

With that, the lesson ended. I had always known about the connection of all life on our planet but The Lord put the connection together in such a simple, yet profound way that for the first time, I really understood the concept. I am merely relating this interaction here so that you might understand it too.

The Mutual Agreement

Sam had been shopping at the shopping club store for several years. The store charged an annual membership fee. Only members were allowed to shop there. There was always one worker at the entrance asking everyone who wanted to enter to show a membership card. There was another worker at the exit of the store asking everyone who left to show their receipt.

Almost every time Sam went shopping at the store he flowed these two simple rules, he showed his membership card upon entering and he showed his receipt upon leaving. There had been several times that Sam didn't to bother showing his member card upon entering the store and none of the workers who were manning the entrance at the time ever harassed him about it. There were a few times when he didn't show the person at the exit his receipt. No one ever stopped him or said anything to him.

On this particular day, Sam was in a hurry He needed to pick up some of the ingredients necessary to cook breakfast and he needed to go to the store, buy the ingredients, go home and cook breakfast before his older son went off to work. He had to do all of this in the space of 45 minutes. Sam got to the store, picked up the ingredients, stood at the checkout line and paid for the ingredients all within 23 minutes. Then he encountered an obstacle.

When he went to leave, there was a humongous line at the store exit. It was so long he couldn't even see the store exit. Sam peeked his head around towards the other side of the exit door. He saw another worker standing on the other side with just two people waiting to show him their receipt. Sam broke from the line and began running towards the side of the exit with a smaller line.

As he took his first few steps, he saw one of the people in line leaving. The worker started looking at the receipt of the last person in his line. Sam ran faster. Just as he got near the worker at the exit, the worker walked away. Sam, now about 15 feet from the exit door on the side where the worker was standing, stopped walking. He just stood there, trying to figure out what he should do.

Within seconds, another person stopped behind him. Sam looked back at the line that he had stood in before. It was even longer than it was when he got into it. He looked at his watch. Another two minutes had passed. He looked 15 feet in front of him at the head of the long line. He saw one, elderly man slowly and carefully looking at someone's receipt. Sam knew that he didn't want to get back into that long line but now there was no one to look at his receipt on the side of the exit door that he was standing on.

Suddenly, the person standing behind Sam ran around him and out of the exit door on the side they were both standing on. The elderly worker didn't say anything as the man ran out the exit door. Someone in the long line began to yell.

"Really, you're going to leave without showing your receipt?" Said the person in the line.

"I only have a few things. I don't need anyone to look at my receipt." Said the man as he exited the store.

Sam looked back at the long line. Then he followed the man out the exit door. No one said anything to him. As he walked through the parking lot, he felt a little guilty but he really needed to get home and start cooking breakfast. He got to his car and began putting the ingredients into his trunk. Suddenly, he felt a tap on his shoulder. He turned to find a 6' 3" tall, 240 pound, middle aged man standing behind him.

"Where do you get off leaving the store without having your receipt checked?" He asked with an angry scowl on his face.

Sam knew from his voice that he was the same man who yelled at the man who exited the store before he did. He thought about how he would respond to this person who was upset by someone violating the sense of order created by everyone following the rules.

"I have to get home and cook breakfast so my son can eat before he goes to work today and I couldn't wait in that long line or he would have to leave without eating breakfast." Sam said.

"I understand." Said the man. "But we need order to have a society. We cannot have order unless everyone mutually agrees to obey the rules, even if obeying the rules means personal sacrifice for the individual." He continued.

"I can see your point when it comes to obeying laws but this is not a law this is a rule imposed by a private company, which isn't even strictly enforced by the company." Sam replied.

"It starts with disobeying company rules and then running stop signs and then, before you know it, we live in a chaotic, disorderly society!" The man replied. "You sir, are an agent of chaos!" He continued as he walked away.

As Sam drove away he didn't think of himself as an agent of chaos but just as a man who needed to feed his son before he went to work. Then thought of his son, the son he was rushing home to cook breakfast for. His son never seemed to fit into society. He was never orderly. He didn't think within the box, he thought outside the box. He barely passed his classes in high school and couldn't get a job, so he started his own business.

When he did, Sam lent him the money to start it because banks followed the rules and lent money on collateral, not on potential. Everyone else Sam's son knew told him he was crazy or that his business plans wouldn't work. The opinions of those you care about create a mutual agreement all their own, the public perception that you will fail.

Sam believed in his son. To his credit, Sam's son believed in himself and his plans enough to think beyond what everyone else told him. In time, he was successful and his success allowed him to employ three thousand people. Sam's son told him that rules and laws can succeed only by mutual agreement but that sometimes you have to opt out of rules that hold you back in order to pioneer your own path.

The man who confronted Sam at his car thought he was teaching Sam a lesson. Sam did learn something from the man. Not that we must all obey the rules no matter what the personal cost but that the mutual agreements members of society make can make for an orderly society but they can also stop us from realizing our full potential.

How the Way You Act Affects Your Environment

If you take a skipping stone and skip it across a lake, the water ripples. Just as the stone affects the water in the lake, you affect the environment around you by the way you interact it. In fact, how you act creates the environment around you. Here are two examples of this from my life that happened to me recently.

The first one happened while I was standing in line at the grocery store, I observed a man leave his cart in the checkout line. He went to the next aisle to get something he forgot. A lady passed by him and walked over to the line the man had just left. Within seconds, seeing no one there the lady moved his cart away and jumped ahead of him in line. The man returned within fifteen seconds and by then, the woman had already put four things on the conveyer belt. The man asked the woman why she moved his cart and jumped in front of him. The woman replied that he wasn't there so he lost his place. The man and woman got into an argument. Other people in the market watched and as the argument escalated so did the tension in the air. Soon other people began arguing about who was right and who was wrong in the argument between the man and woman.

The second one happened later that same day, I was in line at a chain restaurant. I had a coupon sheet with several coupons and was asking if it was still good, as I believed that day was the last day before the coupons expired. There was a man behind me who had to wait a little longer because of my extended interaction with the cashier. After I gave the cashier the coupon I selected from the sheet I turned to the man who had been standing behind me and apologized for his delay. I offered my coupon sheet to him so he could also take advantage of a coupon if he found something he liked. He used a coupon on the sheet. Then he handed the sheet to the woman standing behind him in line and she also used a coupon on the sheet. They both became more animated and struck up and conversation with each other and with me.

My actions made both of those people smile and changed the environment from isolation to friendly. This is something anyone can do. Anyone can pass on a coupon sheet that is about to expire and offer it to their fellow customers without expecting anything in return. You might consider doing this some time and see if it changes the environment around you.

One Small Candle

VERSE 1
She lived in the middle of the city
But felt like she was living in hell
She wondered how she ended up here
And felt dread as the night fell
She felt so isolated
And scarred by broken dreams
She fell asleep serenaded by
Gunshots, moans and screams
They lit one small candle
And put it next to her window
To fight against the darkness
And let the world know
That one small candle
One soul to stand for right
One small candle
To keep away the night

As she struggled every day
To walk towards her goals while surrounded by
Those who lost their way
She was assaulted by temptations
Hammered by neglect
But kept on walking anyway
One step following the next
She lit one small candle

This went on for years
And things got better over time
She struggled every day
And lit a candle every night
One night before turning in
She looked out and to her surprise
Saw 10,000 other candles
Drowning the darkness with their light

They lit one small candle
And put it next to her window
To fight against the darkness
And let the world know
That one small candle
One soul to stand for right
One small candle
To keep away the night

The End is (not) Near

The times in which we currently live are not the end. They are not even the beginning of the end. They are, however, the end of the beginning. Many false prophets have appeared before humankind proclaiming gloom and doom. They cultivate a handful of followers and often coax them to give up their worldly possessions or even their lives. What a waste.

In truth, humanity is closer to the beginning of its tenure on earth than it is to the end. So, all of humankind's excuses for not trying very hard, for polluting the planet, for ignoring or causing disease and catastrophes are pointless. You're stuck with this planet for some time to come. If the air stinks like rotting garbage, the water is viscous and foul, the earth so depleted of nutrients that it yields scrawny, malnourished crops, it's the air you and your future generations will breathe, the water you and they will drink and the soil you and they will sew and the crops you and they will reap.

There is also no need to fear The Lord. Therefore, there is no need to fear hell fire or the boogeyman or anything else coming to make you pay for keeping that library book a couple of days too long. There is no need to do the right thing because you fear that God is going to get you if you don't. Do the right thing because it is the right thing to do. Do the right thing because it may be an opportunity to act as an Agent of The Lord. Do the right thing because it can help propel humanity towards a brighter future and away from the bad air, viscous water and scrawny crop gloom and doom scenario that could come to pass if you don't.

Because The Lord does not judge you directly, but through the piece of Spiritual DNA that is in you, you have an opportunity to exercise the freedom to truly love The Lord and all of creation. You can choose to take advantage of all the wonderful things on this planet, and to live responsibly to ensure that they are around for your lifetime and those of future generations. You can choose to help others instead of just yourself.

In our lifetimes, humanity will begin a shift in thinking, especially in their perception of The Lord. This will begin as a small, possibly insignificant trickle, but over time shall build into a wave on consciousness that sweeps over all of humanity. This shift, when complete, will signal the end of the beginning period and will usher in the beginning of the middle period of humankind's existence.

When the end does come, it will not come as a shout but as a whisper. It will come over a long period of time, as a byproduct of everything that came before it. It will come as a logical successive link in a chain of events that silently evolved before it. Many people read revelations as if it evolves in the span of a two hour action movie. Read it again as if it evolves over a very long period of time. Think of the symbolism as representing things that humankind has done to our planet out of neglect.

Hope Is The Answer

VERSE 1
Man is an employee
Working and sweating every single day
Doesn't have much money
Still he's got bills to pay
He questions the master
And has a long wait for his reply
Just when He's going to give up
Comes the revelation
That hope is the answer
When all else fades away
VERSE 2
Woman is a mother
She's got a lot of mouths to feed
Feels like a martyr
Frustration is what she bleeds
So many disappointments
Yet her faith it keeps her strong
Kids need someone to look up to
In times of desperation
Hope is the answer
VERSE 3
So much suffering and heartache
Bourne upon this worldly plain
So many caught up in it
That can't see beyond their pain
Cries the Wisdom of the ages

All wounds are healed in time
Like a beacon to the future
Shines the inspiration
That Hope is the answer

We Can Do It

VERSE 1
Talking about things won't get them done
Nothing's happening until the work's begun
The attitude of "Yes We Can"
Works best when you've got a plan

BRIDGE
Positive Motivation
Is the life spark of an enlightened generation
Positive Motivation
Is the life force of an enlightened generation
Positive Motivation
Is the life blood of an enlightened generation

CHORUS
We can do it
All we have to do is make up our minds
We can do it
If we take the time to organize

VERSE 2
Nothing's solved by running away
Face the problem don't be afraid
Correct it quickly cause once it's gone
The path is clear for moving on
BRIDGE
Positive Motivation
Is the life spark of an enlightened generation
Positive Motivation
Is the life force of an enlightened generation

Positive Motivation
Is the life blood of an enlightened generation

CHORUS
We can do it
All we have to do is make up our minds
We can do it
If we take the time to organize

Chapter 4 The Power of Life Lessons in Times of Crisis

What if the purpose of life is to learn what it has to teach us?

What if the obstacles and setbacks we experience are only tests meant to make us stronger?

What if the failures we experience are only meant to teach us what not to do in the future?

What if we are meant to learn, not only from the mistakes we make but also from the mistakes of others?

What if every life experience, no matter how brief or pointless it seems on the surface contains a deeper meaning in the lessons it can yield from the knowledge gained and lessons taught both to the spirit experiencing that life and to the rest of humanity and the universe?

Knowing this, would pain and suffering be purposeless or meaningless?

If the purpose of life is to learn what it has to teach us…

What have you learned?

Life Lessons

"Life is a never ending series of lessons."

The Lord speaks volumes to each of us. Most of us never listen. There are many times in our lives that we are given opportunities to learn life lessons. Sometimes they are presented to us as things that are told to us, seen by us or that happen to us. We are meant to learn from them. Life lessons, however, go beyond our own experience. We must also learn from the experiences of others. We often see people, some that we know, others that we do not know, making mistakes. We are meant to learn from their mistakes as well.

Someone you know might say or do something that has dire consequences for them. Sometimes the event that befalls them is the crescendo of a series of bad decisions and stupid, impulsive acts. Other times, it is the result of one catastrophically bad decision or act. The child who touches the hot stove and burns their hand, the teenager who beats another and ends up in jail or the adult who drives drunk and runs over somebody all should learn a lesson themselves but so should those around them. In the grand scheme of things, sometimes people who suffer dire consequences are meant to serve as an example and / or a warning for others. Those who do not learn from others mistakes may be bound to repeat them. Those who learn from the mistakes of others may be saved from the consequences that befall others.

As each person is supposed to learn from their mistakes, so too are communities of people. Whether these communities are neighborhoods, cities or nations, they must learn from their mistakes and the mistakes of others. The mistakes of ourselves and others have been handed down for millennia in the form of oral and written histories. There is a direct correlation between mistakes made by communities (many of them now extinct) in the past and what communities in the present and future do. Knowing the history of your own people as well as that of other people can broaden your community's horizons and can provide more possibilities for solving problems. There are many peoples in this world but in reality there is but one race, the human race. Humans must learn from the mistakes of the human race and not be confined to studying the trials and tribulations of one segment of it.

So study. Study people and events in your daily life. Study events in the local, national and international news. Study the histories of various cultures. The lessons are there for you to learn from. The broader your education is, the more well- rounded your knowledge and experience is. The broader your education, the more enriched is the Soul you return to The Lord.

The Lesson

A high school teacher decided to teach his student the work ethic. He arranged to have the student help him dig a couple of small trenches in a local park. On the appointed day, they went to the park. The teacher took a shovel he was carrying and briefly showed the student how to dig a small trench. Then he asked the student to dig one. The student complied. When the student finished digging the trench, the teacher asked him to dig another and still another after that. After the student had finished digging several small trenches he stopped. He asked the teacher a question.

"Why am I doing all of the work and you are just watching?" He asked the teacher.

"That is because I am supervising you." replied the teacher.

After another hour had passed and the student had dug several more small trenches, the teacher told him to stop.

"What did you learn from today?' He asked the student.

"I learned the meaning of a new word." replied the student.

"Is the word work?" The teacher asked in eager anticipation.

"No, "said the student the word is supervisor.

"Supervisor?" asked the teacher with a puzzled look on his face.

"Yes," said the student.

"Supervisor, I do all the work, you just watch and you get paid more than me, supervisor." The student continued

The Nature of Suffering and Sacrifice

"Suffering and sacrifice can teach lessons that can lead to enlightenment."

Suffering is a state of being which is accentuated by one's emotional state of being and / or ego. Life will present many opportunities for suffering but suffering is only as bad as you allow it to be. Suffering can be either minimized or intensified by how you react to it.

Suffering is a part of life. It is meant to build character. In these times, it often builds bitterness, resentment and hatred. Suffering can be your greatest teacher if you know how to learn from it. It is through suffering that you learn what you don't like and have an opportunity to make the changes that will eliminate the suffering. Listen to your suffering, analyze what is its cause and work on correcting the cause.

Suffering is also a state of mind. Pain can be very real but there are two types of pain, physical and mental/emotional. The mind and spirit can minimize and sometimes eliminate them both. The annals of history are filled with those who have gone into a trance state and been able to overcome physical pain. Mental and emotional pain can also be overcome. Life is filled with setbacks, disasters and accidents. Many have a certain proclivity towards wallowing in self pity. This only lengthens the time and effect of the suffering. Focusing on potential solutions instead of focusing on crying about the problem can help minimize suffering.

In the grand scheme of things, suffering is meant to teach a lesson. Whether the lesson is meant for an individual, a group, a culture, a nation or a planet depends on the suffering. The nature of suffering is that it shall continue until the lesson is learned. Sometimes it takes a lot of repeating until the lesson is learned. Both good and bad people reap the benefits of the sunshine. Both good and bad people receive rain for their crops. Chaos and disaster befalls both the good and the bad. The difference in the aftermath of tragedy is the lesson learned or not learned. The nature of suffering is that it shall continue until the lesson is learned. This is true for an individual, a community, a nation or a planet.

Sacrifice is denying oneself something for the purpose of advancing forward towards a planned outcome or goal. This can work for an individual goal (like atonement or spiritual enlightenment), a familial goal (saving money for your child's college, stopping smoking so you can live long enough to see your child go to college) or a community goal (like cutting down on pollution through recycling).

Sacrifice is also meant to build character. It also teaches lessons. Beyond this, sacrifice helps achieve goals. It has an end product which is tangible. Going without something or with less of something one day, could mean that it will be available another day. This speaks directly towards conserving resources whether they are resources of the individual or of the planet.

While there is rarely a need for suffering (other than catharsis, building character or teaching a lesson), and suffering can be minimized by ones personal outlook, there is often a need for sacrifice. People who squander what they have over a short period of time or who act as gluttons, hoarding and pigging out on resources often end up resourceless or friendless or both. Life is a long haul. It takes sacrifice to make it to the finish line.

People who do not sacrifice often become selfish. Communities who do not sacrifice often find themselves out of resources. Societies who do not sacrifice, rarely achieve anything worth noting.

Reputation

Your reputation
Is what you think you are
In a galaxy of people
You can be a shining star
Your reputation
It can make you
Or it can break you

Your reputation
Is what other people see
It's their way of making you
Into what they want you to be
You can be broken
By words spoken
By your reputation

Your reputation
Can push you ahead
It can give you wings of gold
Or feet of lead
Your reputation
It can make you
Or it can break you

Your reputation
Is based upon your actions
It loses its grip
If you don't give satisfaction
You can be broken
By words spoken
By your reputation

A Blessing in Disguise

Have you ever had something bad happen to you, only to find out later that it was actually a blessing in disguise? Bad things happen to good people all the time but it while some hold on to the pain caused by bad things like it was a precious jewel, allowing that pain to hold them back from trying new experiences, others let it go and move forward with their lives.

It has been written that everything happens for a reason. It is true, everything does happen for a reason it's just that the person it is happening to often doesn't know what the reason was at the time things are happening to them. The reason usually only becomes clear in hindsight, after the incident has long passed and some perspective can be achieved.

So, what is the difference between the people who are devastated by the bad things that happen to them and those who seem to move beyond the trauma associated with the incident quickly? The people who move on quickly are often people in one of three categories: they are people of faith, spiritual people or people with a positive outlook.

People of faith often move beyond the bad things that happen to them because they have been taught through their religion that God watches over and protects them. They have a holy book, filled with stories and parables which illustrate this point. They have religious authorities that they can go to for guidance. They have a community of people who believe as they do, who they can count on for support. They move forward with the help of other people of faith as a member of a caring community.

Spiritual people believe in a higher power. They believe that higher power is ultimately good and that bad things are a part of life. They seek to learn the lesson that the bad thing was sent to teach them. They move forward because they know that the bad thing that just happened to them happened for a reason. They may not know the reason just yet but knowing that it happened for a reason gives them the strength to move forward.

People with a positive outlook on life may not have religion. They may not even believe in higher power. They are strengthened by their honest belief that good things can come out of bad and that every cloud has a silver lining. They may also be bolstered by thoughts of how much worse the bad thing could have been and count themselves as fortunate that the bad thing wasn't a worse thing. They may also believe that something better is just around the corner. They move forward to get to that something better.

Are you in any of the three groups described above? Do you have a holy book, religious authorities and a community behind you? Do you believe that everything happens for a reason and search for the lesson in the event? Do you believe that every cloud has a silver lining? Or...are you a combination of two or more of these three types? If so, congratulations, you have evolved a coping strategy for the bad things that happen in life. If you do not fall into one of the three categories mentioned, what is your coping strategy? How has it been working for you?

Do you let the bad things that happen to you hold you back or do you move forward beyond them? The next time something bad happens to you and trust me, something bad will happen to you sooner or later, remember the type of people that move beyond the bad things that happen to them and see what you can use that will work for you.

The Lizard

I hadn't seen one for about ten years

It seemed alien to the concrete and asphalt world

I was familiar with

Crouching on the pavement, sunning itself

At first, I thought it was one of those toy ones

The kind that bratty little brothers leave on their sister's

pillow

But as I bent down to pick it up

It moved

I lunged forward and grabbed it

As I held it firmly in my grip

I noticed that it looked scaly

But was smooth to the touch

It began squirming

I wanted to take it home

But its squirming became more violent with each step I

took

I wanted to make it my pet

To take care of it

But somehow, in its squirming

I could sense its strong desire to be free

Free where cats could pounce on it

Free where cars could run over it

Free where people could step on it

Deep in a concrete jungle

Miles away from the nearest mountain

I let it go

The Secret of Spiritual Growth

There are trials and tribulations in every life. There is sickness and disability. There are scars that heal slowly and scars that never heal completely. There is loneliness, loss and all manner of suffering. There is frustration and failure. There are dreams that are deferred and dreams that are never realized. It is not the defeats in life that defeat you but how you react to them. Those who learn the lessons that can be yielded from these experiences will minimize their effect and use them to become more than they were before they happened.

For in reality they are merely lessons. They may be hard lessons but they are merely lessons nonetheless. It is life's bitter moments that make its pleasant moments sweet. It is life's struggles that make the successes seem worthwhile. It is the difficulty of the uphill climb that gives the downhill coasting its full pleasure. It is the effort put into something that gives it its true value.

So let the trials and tribulations come; you can withstand them. Let sickness and disability nip at your body and slow you down; your spirit will propel you forward. Let the scars remind you, not of what you have lost but of what you have triumphed over. Let the loss and loneliness change what you value and let the suffering strengthen you. Let the frustration and failure teach you what not to do and make room for the wisdom that shows you what to do. Let them nag at you until you move beyond them into the next phase of your journey. Let the dreams deferred and never realized be replaced with dreams that can be realized.

Author Biographies

Author Biography

Mark Wilkins

A Storyteller

My name is Mark Wilkins. I am best known to my readers as A Storyteller. I pen the A Storyteller Series of Books for Love Force International Publishing. Unlike most other book series, it does not concentrate on a particular character or a particular story line. Instead, it focuses on books of short stories in various genres by a particular author, namely myself. Some of the books in the A Storyteller Book Series include serious fiction (A Week's Worth of Fiction), humorous fiction (Slices of Life) and a mixture of serious and humorous fiction and non-fiction (Classroom Confessions) and supernatural Fiction (Stories of The Supernatural).

The readers who enjoy my books like reading that sparks their imagination. They like stories with memorable and quirky characters on unusual topics. They like unexpected twists and turns in the plot. If any of these things my readers enjoy describe you, then you too will enjoy my writing.

I am comfortable writing in many different genres. I write both humorous and serious fiction. Some of my stories are based on true events, others are totally my invention. It is up to you, the reader, to decide which stores are based on factual events and which are completely my invention because I'm not telling. I like to tell stories and I work very hard at making those stories both compelling and entertaining. I hope you enjoy reading my books.

Author Biography

The Prophet of Life

I am a journalist, author and songwriter. I write the Faith and Spiritual books as well as topical, thematic literature books for Love Force International Publishing.

I have had very broad and varied life experiences and those experiences enrich my writing. I write on Spiritual topics as well as topics of global importance. I write non-fiction that tells it like it is but that is solution oriented as opposed to just complaining about things. I have books on topics such as Crime and Punishment, Racism, and Faith.

I like writing things from unique perspectives. I like to challenge my reader's perceptions and allow them to come away with new insights. If a lesson can be woven into the fabric of the written word, so much the better but the lesson is often subtle.

I try and see things the way they are and the way that they can be. This allows me to see the possibilities within various situations both in my life and in the things I write. As a result, I can often add twists and turns readers will not likely see coming in fiction I write. I can often communicate things from unique and different perspectives and see solutions to problems and issues that I communicate about in my nonfiction.

I am not afraid to take risks both in my life and in my writing. I have tackled controversial issues in both. My nonfiction Word Press blog, Insight, a blog by The Prophet of Life, is full of examples. I have an offbeat sense of humor and have written humorous things as well as serious. I started a You Tube Channel and now have over 100 videos that have words and music but no pictures. Despite the fact that there are no pictures over 150,000 people from 210 different nations have viewed the videos on my You Tube channel.

I enjoy hearing from my readers. I enjoy writing. I hope you will find my books interesting and entertaining.

Author Bio

DR Goose

My name is Dr. Goose. I have been working with children of all ages for over 30 years. I would describe my writing style as descriptive enough to give children a basic idea of what the characters look like while sparking their imagination to fill in the details. My books are specifically designed to help children develop their imaginations.

My stories take children to exciting new places which are a composite of blended cultures. I try to make my characters and the settings in my stories exciting and different. I also try and give them enough familiarity to provide a foundation upon which children can paint their own mental pictures of the setting and characters in the stories.

I write stories for children of all ages. It is important for parents to read the age ranges for each book. Doing so will help to insure their child is reading a book appropriate to their developmental level.

In our modern, technologically advanced world, children have everything done for them, in books, on T.V., in movies and in electronic gaming and as a result, they have difficulty with creativity. Developing one's imagination is a benchmark for developing creativity. My books are designed to develop a child's imagination. I suggest that parents who wish to help their child in this process provide paper and colored pencils or crayons and ask their child to draw what they think the characters or setting look like. This will help children develop their imaginations and creativity even further.

Kindle Books by Love Force International Publishing

Whether you are interested in true stories, fiction, humor, action, adventure, spiritual insights, quotes, poetry, self-help or children's books, Love Force International has got you covered. **Our 99-cent commitment,** our commitment to a 99 cent price for all our kindle e book titles so that people around the globe can afford them, means there has never been a better time to stock up on Books published by Love Force International!

Love Force International Publishing Company is a full-service publishing company which is committed to offering a wide selection of literature at affordable prices. All of our e-books are 99 cents. All of our paperbacks are at least 100 pages in length. Most range from $6.50 to $9.00. We offer a wide variety of literature in different formats and languages. A complete list of our paperbacks is at the end of this section. We offer both e-books and Paperbacks. We offer books in English and books in Spanish. We offer both fiction & non-fiction. We offer Literature for all ages from children to adult. We offer literature in various genres, including: Action & Adventure, Humor, Dystopic, Ethnic, Children's, (from very young to Juvenile) Mystical, Occult, Horror, Spiritual and Religious as well as Poetry. We offer non-fiction in various genres including True Crime, Inspirational, Global Issues, Self Help and even Quotes. Our books are available as e-books and in print through Amazon Kindle exclusively.

Many of our books have informational videos on Amazon. These videos give you insight into how the author created the book. The videos are on both the book pages and the author pages. Some of the contents in our books are available in other formats including video with audio. These are available on You Tube for FREE. You can find them by typing the name of the channel into google. Some of our humorous content can be found on Randomand Anonymous. Some of our spiritual and topical content can be found on: the true prophet of life You Tube channel but you need to type all of the words: the true prophet of life together in this fashion in order to access it. Many contents of our products can be found on the Loveforce International You Tube channel as well.

NOTE: Books with ASINs are available now the others will be available soon. All Titles are printed in English. Books with an **SP** after the title also have a version translated into Spanish. Our books available in a paperback version books will have **Ppr** on the same line as the title.

The Reader Series is a series of readers that are a sampling of writings by one or more authors.

The Prophet of Life Reader (7 Book Sampler) V 1 & 2
What do essays, articles, stories, poetry and quotes have in common? They are all in this sampling of stories, poems and other writings from 7 of The Prophet of Life's writings found in these Kindle books.
Author: The Prophet of Life   **ISBN:** 978-1-936462-07-0
ASIN: B015D716C0 (Vol 1)   **ASIN:** B06XBSWKX8 (Vol 2)

The Mark Wilkins Reader 7 Book Sampler! Volumes 1 & 2
One story from seven books by Mark Wilkins. Whether its smart spouses, inquisitive fools, teachers, gangsters or ghosts these books give you a good sampling of stories by the man known throughout the world as A Storyteller. Within its pages you will find horror, humor and pathos.
 Author: Mark Wilkins   **ISBN:** 978-1-936462-38-4
ASIN: B01MU0Z51H **Volume 1**

The Love Force International Reader 7 Book Sampler! 4 Books in This Series
Whether you want fiction, humor, children's stories, poetry or quotes these books have got all of those and more! A sampling of 7 different books by three authors offered in Kindle books published by Love Force International.
Edited by Evan Lovefire   **Vol 1 ASIN:** B06XBHD9RX
Vol 2 ASIN: B06XBMGLNK
Vol 3 ASIN: B07DCGTLKF   **Vol 4**
ASIN: B07DP51BWG

The Love Force International Sampler, Spanish Books Edition SP Volumes 1 2, 3, 4
In The Loveforce International Sampler series each book contains a sampling of 7 different books by three or four different authors. The first two books in the series are translated into Spanish. **(Edited by** C. Gomez) Vol 1 **ASIN: B06XB3RJ2K Vol 2 ASIN:**

The True Stories Series is a series of books which include true stories by The Prophet of Life.

True Stories!   SP

A riveting collection of true stories. Whether you want to know about the toddler taken by a gator at a Disney Resort, an 18 year old who doesn't exist, which popular restaurant chain has a corporate mentality of public humiliation for its employees or an alarming new trend that could affect your household this book has got it all and they are all absolutely true!

Author: The Prophet of Life   **ISBN: 978-1-936462-16-2**
ASIN: B06XVSZSZ9

True Stories: Inspiration and General Interest
SP

What do cell phone addicts, George Orwell, birds, Paul McCartney, The Nobel Prize, Black Friday, Led Zeppelin, garbage, a pep talk, tipping, Steve Jobs, Shakespeare, inspirational thoughts and your mother have in common? They are in true stories in this book. True Stories of Inspiration & General Interest brings together stories and poems about celebrities, trends and everyday people. Sometimes surprising, always interesting, it will entertain you and give you something to think about at the same time.

Author: The Prophet of Life   **ISBN: 978-1-936462-15-5**
ASIN: B00TXWVNUC   ASIN: B01BBCKFZU
(Spanish Edition)

Controversy

Ppr SP

What do Caitlyn Jenner, Donald Trump, a cure for AIDS, Chinese hackers, Adolf Hitler and Global Warming have in common? They are all at the heart of a controversy and there are stories about them in this unique book that turns tabloid headlines inside out.

Author: The Prophet of Life **ISBN:** **978-1-936462-19-3 ASIN: B016MWU8NS ASIN: B01CRF3098 (Spanish Edition)**

True Stories of Crime and Punishment

SP

This book of serious crime stories is ripped from headlines all over the globe. From the family that vanished, to the 11 year old girl killed in a fight over a boy, to the prisoner who hasn't eaten in 14 years, to the severed human head found near the famous Hollywood sign these stories ripped will astound you and give you pause to think.

Author: The Prophet of Life **ISBN: 978-1-936462-17-9 ASIN: B01406YZBE ASIN: B01N10ND7S (Spanish Edition)**

Strange but True!

A collection of facts and stories about people, places and things that are strange and seem like fiction but are absolutely true!

Author: Mark Wilkins **ISBN: ASIN:**

The A Storyteller Series is a unique book series. Instead of concentrating on a particular character or genre, the series consists of collections of short stories by Author Mark Wilkins, Also Known As A Storyteller.

Slices of Life Volume 1 Ppr* SP
is a collection of humorous short stories about life. Most of them deal with marriage and family members. From smart spouses to intelligent little children to guys trying to impress their friends and in-laws trying to master technology each story is like a little slice of life but together, they make up an irresistible pie. Sit back, grab a cup of coffee and enjoy some slices of lie because, before you know it, you will have finished the whole thing.
Author: Mark Wilkins **ISBN: 978-1-936462-11-7**
ASIN: B014ZF5VY0   ASIN: B01BBBZUL0
(Spanish Edition)

Slices of Life Volume 2 Ppr* SP
This sequel to Slices of Life has more humorous stories about the rich, the poor and the middle class. It even has a story about one of their pets. Ignorance is the main theme of this book, ignorance that has consequences that are sometimes touching but always humorous. So brew so coffee or tea, sit down and relax and enjoy another satisfying batch of more slice of life because, before you know it, you will have devoured the whole thing.
Author: Mark Wilkins **ISBN: 978-1-936462-12-4 ASIN: B01M2B3YZ1 ASIN: B06XKP5C66   (Spanish Edition)**

*Slices of Life Volumes 1 &2 combined are available in Paperback In English under Slices of Life ISBN-13: 978-1936462452 and in Spanish under Rabanadas de Vida ISBN-13: 978-1936462469

Stories of The Supernatural Volume 1 Ppr* SP
Ghosts, demonic creatures, and Death. This collection of Short Stories will haunt and entertain you. Whether it's the classic evil of A Lump of Coal or the whimsy of A Ghost in the House this collection of Short Stories and poems will haunt, thrill and entertain you.
Author: Mark Wilkins **ISBN: 9781936462186 ASIN: B01M1N1QR5 ASIN: B01MA12YXY (Spanish Edition)**

Stories of The Supernatural Volume 2 Ppr* SP
In this sequel to Stories of The Supernatural there are more Ghosts, Demonic Creatures and Death. This collection of short stories Centers of Ghosts and Monsters. Within its pages you will marvel at the exploits of The Soul Collector, Shudder at the mention of the dreaded Bungadun and of the Hell Banger and ride the rails on the ghost train. Strap on your seat belts, it's going to be a bumpy ride! **Author:** Mark Wilkins
ISBN: 9781936462261 ASIN: B01MDJMSUY ASIN: B01M4FXDL1 (Spanish Edition)

*A Paperback version of Stories of the Supernatural 1 & 2 combined is available in both English and Spanish. The English is under the same title ISBN-13: 978-1936462537And the Spanish paperback edition is entitled Historias Sobrenaturales, ISBN-13: 978-1936462575.

A Week's Worth of Fiction: Volume 1
Ppr*   SP
In Volume 1 of A Week's Worth of Fiction, People on The Edge, you will meet people on the edges of society. A security guard who struggles with a dying wife, an elderly man whose cast aside and left to die, one woman struggling to capture romance before her beauty fades and another struggling with cancer. You will meet a little boy who terrorizes a grocery store, a teenage boy searching for love and a small businessman struggling against a monopoly. If you want fictional stories you will never forget you only need to count to 7.**Author:** Mark Wilkins **ISBN: 978-1-936462-13-1 ASIN: B01521SQ02 ASIN: B06XVD21PM (Spanish Edition)**

A Week's Worth of Fiction Volume 2
Ppr* SP
Volume 2 of A Week's Worth of Fiction, Science Fiction you will be intrigued and astounded by stories about a girl who has the cure for a deadly disease, a woman on a date with psycho somatic disease called prophecy, a robot chicken, a supernatural fly, an astral projection, a teacher in a new job where everything is not what it seems and a futuristic world where the only economy is barter. If you want science fiction stories you will never forget you only need to count to 7.

Author: Mark Wilkins   **ISBN: 9781936462148 ASIN:** B01LX9RZH7   **ASIN:** B071GCYFK6   (**Spanish Edition**)

* A Week's Worth of Fiction Volumes 1 & 2 are combined in an available paperback in English under the title A Week's Worth of Fiction Volumes 1&2 With an ISBN-13: 978-1936462551.

A Week's Worth of Fiction Volume 3
     SP
A Week's Worth of Fiction Volume 3, The Many Sides of Violence, features 7 fictional stories that explore violence. One story looks at what goes through the mind of a terrorist about to blow himself up. Another, looks at an executive considering suicide. The plots of other stories include a, man trying to outwit an armed carjacker, a sky marshal trying to figure out which passage is a terrorist, a soldier who realizes someone in his platoon is a serial killer, an ex-convict who has to decide if he should use violence to combat evil and an everyman who becomes a hero through unspeakable violence, if you want violent stories you will never forget you only need to count to 7.
Author: Mark Wilkins   **ASIN: B071WNC6ZX   ASIN:** B072K6J9HN   (**Spanish Edition**)

A Week's Worth of Fiction Volume 4
     SP

In A Week's Worth of Fiction 4, Realizations, you will meet people from various backgrounds who come to important realizations. You will meet a Doctor who comes to a realization about old age, a politician who struggles to be his own man, a rich man who reaches an epiphany after a chance encounter at a store, A farmer in need of help, A little boy who struggles with a new cell phone that seems processed, a swimmer who gains insight from her morning routine and a police officer who develops empathy for a hardcore gangster. If you want the fictional stories you will never forget you only need to count to 7.

Author: Mark Wilkins   **ASIN: B07217QL6H**
ASIN: B071JVQQ96   (Spanish Edition)

Classroom Confessions Volume 1
Ppr*   SP
is a series of true stories from the front lines of public education. Within its pages you will meet quirky characters, the good, the bad and the over caffeinated. Some of them are teachers, some students and some are administrators. Some will make you laugh, others will make you cry but they all play an important role in public education. Their stories are written in way that will entertain you and give you something to think about.
Author: Mark Wilkins **ISBN: 978-1-936462-08-7**
ASIN: B00VNFJBX8   ASIN: B01MSV4N92
(Spanish Edition)

Classroom Confessions Volume 2
Ppr* SP

Is another series of true stories from the front lines of public education. Within its pages you will meet unforgettable characters like the French Substitute, Mr. Happyhands, Harry Winkwater, The Bushwhacker and of course, Julian. Some will touch your heart, others will give you something to think about but they will all entertain you. **Author:** Mark Wilkins   **ASIN: B01N1OCRVC ASIN: B06XC9HDQV (Spanish Edition)** *Classroom Confessions volumes 1 & 2 combined are available in paperback as Public School Confessions, ISBN-13: 978-1936462056. And in Spanish as Confesiones de Escuelas Publicas, ISBN-13: 978-1936462063.

The Love Force Novella Series: These are short novels of varying length.
Karma   Ppr   SP
The story of one man who negotiates between two different cultures, and opposing life views competing for his attention. His conflicts and struggles are overshadowed by cosmic forces he cannot understand. Karma provides insights into the struggles and conflicts we all face.
Author: Mark Wilkins
ASIN: B0722R448R (English Edition) ASIN: B072Z6L36V (Spanish Edition) Paperback English: ISBN-13: 978-1936462506
Paperback in Spanish: ISBN-13: 978-1936462582

The Beyond Faith Series
Is a series of books that look at life from a spiritual
perspective. No matter what your faith, you will find
spiritual insights in these books that will enrich your life.
What Faith Has Taught Me
Ppr* SP
 I am just an ordinary person who has been privileged to
have a life filled with miracles and revelations. There are
many times when I had nothing except faith but faith was
all I needed to sustain me. My faith and my God have
taught me many life lessons. This book shares some of the
things my faith has taught me and the spiritual insights I
have gained because of my faith.
Author: The Prophet of Life   **ISBN: 978-1-936462-03-2**
ASIN: B01527IKT8   ASIN: B01EE3QSW2
(Spanish Edition)

Finding God in A Chaotic World
     Ppr* SP
The world can seem so chaotic these days. Many people
long for guidance. Many others want to get closer to God.
How do you find God amidst the chaos and confusion?
How can you discern God's messages from the multi-
media blitz we are each bombarded with every day? Some
people are part of an organized religion. Others are
spiritual without a particular religion. Some are still
searching, All of them trying to find God.

In this book, you will learn that The Lord communicates with how The Lord communicates with you. You will learn about the True Nature of God and realize just how profound God's Love and reach are. You will learn the secret of why God's will always prevails. If you are ready for revelations that may change the way you look at life in general and your life in particular, read this book.
Author: The Prophet of Life **ISBN: 978-1-936462-01-8**
ASIN: B00SLLZAAU

Finding God without Religion
    Ppr* SP
People of faith are not exclusive to religion. There are many who are spiritual or agnostic. They don't fit into the doctrine, rituals and congregational community of religion. In this wisdom filled volume, people of faith but without an organized religion can gain insights into life, the afterlife and God without being brow beaten or guilt tripped into conversion. This volume is Book 2 of the Revelations of 2012 Beyond Faith series. Part 1 is entitled Finding God in A Chaotic World.
Author: The Prophet of Life **ISBN: 978-1-936462-10-0**
ASIN: B00XKPD86K

Inspiration For All 1
Ppr* SP
Selected Inspirational Writings. Whether you are of faith or just in need of inspiration in your life, this book full of inspirational stories, poems and essays will sustain and strengthen you on your journey. **Authors: The Prophet of Life & Mark Wilkins ASIN: B071ZM17V6**

Inspiration for All 2
SP
This is a book of selected inspirational writings by three different authors. It will not only entertain you but will also stimulate your mind by offering you alternative ways of looking at things and opportunities to gain insights. **Authors**: Mark Wilkins, The Prophet of Life & Dr. Goose. **ASIN: B0736JH6M9** Spanish **ASIN: B072WK9JBH**

* What Faith Has Taught Me and The Best Quotes about God (ASIN: B018P0M8OC) and Inspiration for All (ASIN: B018P0M8OC) are combined in a paperback edition published in both English and Spanish. In English it is called The Faith Trilogy ISBN-13: 978-1936462513 and in Spanish under the title La trilogia de la fe ISBN-13: 978-1936462520

* Finding God in A Chaotic World, Finding God without Religion and The Best Spiritual Quotes (ASIN: B01MQVA87Q) are combined into one paperback The Agnostic Faith Trilogy ISBN-13: 978-1936462476 and La trilogia Agnostico de la Fe ISBN-13: 978-1936462599 in Spanish.

Outrageous Humor Series
Books of stories and fake news articles for those with an off-beat sense of humor.

Outrageous Stories 1
    Ppr* SP
This book is filled with offbeat humor articles. All of them are fictitious and many of them completely outrageous. No one is safe from being made fun of be they terrorists, Presidents, Dictators, The Movie and Record Business or couch potatoes. If you are college age or older and have an offbeat, irreverent, sense of humor, this book is for you!
Author: Mark Wilkins **ISBN: 978-1-936462-33-9 ASIN: B01LY3VZJR**

More Outrageous Stories
    Ppr* SP
This book is filled with more offbeat humor articles. All of them are fictitious and many of them completely outrageous. No one is safe from being made fun of be they terrorists, Racists, National Holidays or the medical establishment. If you are college age or older and have an offbeat, irreverent, sense of humor, this book is for you!
Author: Mark Wilkins **ISBN: 978-1-936462-33-9 ASIN: ASIN: B074Y8LTTJ**

Outrageous Stories 3
       Ppr*

This book is filled with even more offbeat humor articles. All of them are fictitious and many of them completely outrageous. No one is safe from being made fun of being made fun of including dictators, TV, fashion trends, Shakespeare and new species. If you are college age or older and have an offbeat, irreverent, sense of humor, this book is for you! **Author:** Mark Wilkins
ASIN: B07J9MQSFP

*Outrageous Stories 1, 2 & 3 are combined into the paperback entitled Totally Outrageous Stories! ISBN-13: 978-1936462490

Self Help Series
This consists of books by different authors designed to help people improve their lives.

Becoming The Person You've Always Wanted to Be
SP
This self-help book offers a simple, yet profound method of making positive changes in your life. It includes a link to download exclusive, helpful companion worksheets to help you become the person you have always wanted to be.
Author: Mark Wilkins **ISBN: 978-1-936462-39-1   ASIN: B01MSYVAB6**
            ASIN: B01MSYVU6R   (Spanish Edition)

Life Success Kit
SP
Spiritual Thought Leader The Prophet of Life helps you clarify what success really means to you through a series of inspirational life lessons designed to give you new perspectives on achieving success and a blueprint for making changes in the things that are preventing you from becoming a success.
Author: The Prophet of Life   **ASIN: B01MZ2TSCP**
Spanish Edition: ASIN: B078JZGWDH

The Your Life in Rhyme Poetry Series
Is a series of Poetry books unlike any you have ever read
whether it is an exploration of life itself through a thematic
chapter on each of the various stages of life as in
Reflections in The Mirror of Life, The mixture of thought
provoking essays and inspirational poetry of Black in
America or the exploration of a single topic as in Romance
Returns or Life in Verse. The books in this series will have
you rediscovering poetry in a way that will make you
wonder why you ever avoided it in the first place.

Reflections in the Mirror of Life This unique book explores life through its harsh realities, pleasant diversions and positive possibilities. The book looks at modern society, the problems it faces, and the people who are a part of it. In a unique twist that's different from most books of poetry, Reflections is divided into five chapters, each of which explores a different theme woven into the fabric of modern life. The tone for each chapter is set by a free verse poem which is followed by a series of rhyming poems on that theme.
Author: The Prophet of Life **ISBN: 978-1-936462-04-9 ASIN: B00V2TSAXC**

Black in America is an exploration of racism through essays and poems. It spans from the beginnings of the Civil Rights movement through today. It looks at people who have been lightning rods for race relations in America and has some surprising insights into the people and events that have shaped race relations in America for the past 60 years. This book is a good companion for anyone who wants to gain insight into the Civil Rights movement, race relations and racism itself.   **Author:** The Prophet of Life   **ISBN**: 978-1-936462-09-4   **ASIN: B00S05QSXA**

Every Lyric Tells A Story   SP A collection of unique song lyrics that tell compelling stories about people, their lives, their hopes and dreams. You can find yourself and people you know in many of them.
Author: The Prophet of Life & Mark Wilkins   **ASIN: B01NAFDWZW**

Romance Lives! Romance Lives is a very special collection of Romantic Love Poems. The poems are arranged to follow the arc of a romance from its early, puppy love stages through its sweet seductions and the blissful wisdom of mature love.   If you are searching for Romance in your love relationship or just want some joyful, insightful romantic reading this book is for you! **Authors: The Prophet of Life & Mark Wilkins ISBN: ASIN: B07D9WY6V5**

Life in Verse
A collection of poems about life. The poems and song lyrics are about people, their lives, their hopes and dreams. You can find yourself and people you know in many of them. **Author:** The Prophet of Life **ISBN:**   **ASIN:**

The Best Quotes quotation series
Is a series of books filled with quotes attributed to the
Prophet of Life whose quotes have been used by charities,
corporations, institutions of Medicine and higher learning.
The book includes a license to use any of the quotes as
long as they are attributed to The Prophet of Life.

The Best Quotes About God   **SP**
This short book is filled with some of the more popular
quotes about God attributed to The Prophet of Life. It is
both thought provoking and inspirational. It is filled with
dozens of quotes about God that one can read and copy for
personal use.
Author: The Prophet of Life **ISBN: 978-1-936462-20-9**
ASIN: B018P0M8OC ASIN: B01BJXYHLY
(Spanish Edition)

The Best Quotes on General Subjects
    SP
This short book is filled with some of the more popular
quotes on general subjects attributed to The Prophet of
Life. The book includes quotes on topics such as life, love,
happiness, crime and punishment, wellness and includes
many of the humorous quotes attributed to The Prophet of
Life. You will find the wit and wisdom in its pages thought
provoking and inspirational. It is filled with dozens of
quotes about God that one can read and copy for personal
use. **Author:** The Prophet of Life **ISBN:**
ASIN: B01M58L9LW

The Best Spiritual Quotes
SP

This book is filled with some of the more popular quotes on Spiritual Subjects attributed to The Prophet of Life. Included are quotes on faith, mercy, life lessons, humanity and spirituality. You should find them to be profound, thought provoking and inspirational. It is filled with many pages of quotes that one can read and copy for personal use.

Author: The Prophet of Life   **ASIN**: **B01MQVA87Q**

Children Storybook Series
All books are by Dr. Goose who writes in both prose and rhyming verse.
Classic Children's Stories You've Likely Never Heard SP
Help develop your child's creative abilities and develop their imagination by reading them stories from this book that has no illustrations. Whether it's a story about Prince trying to find the answer to a question, a spider talking about a savior, a kingdom in trouble or a child trying to save the world you will find yourself wanting to read these children's stories with international flavor again and again. This first book in the series is for smaller children.
Author: Dr. Goose **ISBN: 9781936462407 ASIN: B01NAF8QNU ASIN: B01MR5PR84** (Spanish Edition)

More Classic Children's Stories You've Likely Never Heard SP
This sequel gives you more unknown classics. The book introduces new characters like a little chicken whose life is similar to a person's and a ballad about a hairy man. There is a story about a prince whose refusal causes an international incident. There is even an updated version of classic children's story everyone knows from different character's points of view. This second book in the series helps tweens and juvenile children creative abilities and develop their imagination as stories from this book that has no illustrations either.
Author: Dr. Goose **ISBN: 978-1-936462-41-4 ASIN:** **ASIN:** (Spanish Edition)

My First Book of Stupid Little Fables
SP
Whether the greed of mooches and lunch thieves, sadistic children, or bizarre stories about pets this first installment in the series of irreverently humorous stories with twisted endings about the selfish and the greedy delivers. It even has the stupid little drawings! For Juveniles.
 Author: Gary Ishka   **ISBN: 9781936462445**
ASIN:B07GJPJ2CD   ASIN: B07FFF13N4 (Spanish Edition)

My Second Book of Stupid Little Fables   SP
Whether it's well-meaning but incompetent grandmas, egotistical women, sadistic children, or crazy people in shopping centers, this second installment in the series of irreverently humorous stories with twisted endings about the selfish and the greedy delivers. It even has the drawings you love to make fun of just like the first one! For Juveniles.
Author: Dr. Gary Ishka   **ISBN: ASIN:**
          ASIN: (Spanish Edition)

More Children's Stories
School Kidz Volume 1 Elementary and Middle School SP
Six funny stories about kids who are smarter than their age. Within its pages you will meet A boy whose vocabulary is better than the adults in his school, a kid who escapes a spanking, A kid who gets a new cell phone with a built-in problem and a brother and sister who learn how get rid of junk from an old aunt. Recommended for kidz ages 12-16. **Author: Mark Wilkins ASIN: B0717B6SQ4**

School Kidz Volume 2 High School   SP
9 stories about kids who are in high school. Within its pages you will meet a group of Kidz who get involved in a rotten egg war, a girl who doesn't exist, and a kid who sends a friend on a date with his sister. Recommended for kidz ages 14-18. **Author: Mark Wilkins ASIN: B071W5WZZN**

AIRCO Fanbooks
These are recording artist fan books by artists who are members of Affiliated Independent Recording Creators Organizaion (AIRCO).

Teacherz Text Book, The Alternative Lesson Plan Project.
This book is about Alernative Rock band Teacherz their story, their songs and lyrics for songs in the Alternative Lesson Plan Project.
Author: Mark Wilkins ASIN:

Coming Soon E Workbooks and an E Textbook!
A series of mini and one comprehensive E Textbook
Under the title of Mr. Wilkins Teaches English by
Mark Wilkins
The specific mini textbooks will be on topics such as
Reading and Responding to Literature, and Methods for
Writing Paragraphs and Essays. The Comprehensive text
will include a weekly spelling component and both the
mini texts and comprehensive Text will include creative
lessons that promote creativity and critical thinking in
students while fitting into common core standards. The
mini texts will be no more than 99 cents each and the
comprehensive text will be paperback for under $10!
All of the books are freshly created and contain exclusive
intellectual property you won't find in any other texts.
These books are perfect for students learning high school
English levels 9 & 10 whether you are a classroom teacher
or are home schooling your child. We are making the
commitment to keep all of the books at low prices to allow
parents and school districts to afford texts in the face of
shrinking educational budgets. Purchasers will be given an
opportunity to receive an email with a printable version of
the exercises and assignments as well as links to online
testing free of charge.
Author: Mark Wilkins   **ISBN: ASIN:**

Compelling Stories for Adaptation to Short Film
For Film Students
Compelling stories in a set location with six or less
characters. Easily adaptable to screenplay with notes on
adapting them.
Author: Mark Wilkins   **ISBN: ASIN:**

Loveforce International Paperbacks

Most of our paperback books cost between $6.50 and $8.50

Stories of The Supernatural: A Storyteller Series Book SP Loveforce Duo

This collection of 15 stories is filled with ghosts, demonic creatures, monsters and death. It will haunt you, thrill you and entertain you. Within its pages you will marvel at the exploits of The Soul Collector,and the uniqueness of Life Lines and Cannibal Money. You will shudder at the mention of a lump of coal or the dreaded Bungadun of Blood Valley and ride the rails on the ghost train. Strap on your seat belts, it's going to be a bumpy ride! **Author:** Mark Wilkins **ISBN-10: 1936462532 ISBN-13: 978-1936462537**

Karma

Karma is the story of one man who negotiates between two different cultures, and opposing life views competing for his attention. His conflicts and struggles are overshadowed by cosmic forces he cannot understand. Karma provides insights into the struggles and conflicts we all face. **Author: Mark Wilkins ISBN-10:** 1936462508 **ISBN-13:** 978-1936462506   **SP ISBN-10:** 1936462583

A Week's Worth of Fiction Volumes 1 & 2
    Loveforce Duo

Whether it's people on the edges of society or Science
Fiction Stories, this collection of Volumes 1 & 2 of A
Week's Worth of Fiction gives you 2 volumes each with 7
stories that will thrill you, surprise you and make you
think. Often dystopic and sometimes surreal, if you want
stories you will never forget you only need to count to 7
and you can do it twice in this special paperback edition.
**Author: Mark Wilkins ISBN-10: 1936462559 ISBN-
9781936462551**

Totally Outrageous Stories! Outrageous Satire
    Loveforce Trio

There is absolutely nothing that escapes ridicule in this
flagrantly outrageous, biting satire of everything you can
imagine. This smart, flippant book pokes fun at the
entertainment industry, the medical establishment, politics,
societal norms, history and science. If you want to laugh to
humor with no mercy, you have to get totally outrageous!
Author: Mark Wilkins   ISBN-10: 1936462494   **ISBN-
13:** 978-1936462490

Slices of Life: Stories of Humor and Pathos (A Storyteller Series)   SP Loveforce Duo

Slices of Life Slices is a collection of humorous short stories about life. Most of them deal with marriage and family members. There are smart spouses, intelligent little children, guys trying to impress their friends and in-laws trying to master technology. Ignorance is the main theme of this book, ignorance that has consequences that are sometimes touching but always humorous. Each story is like a little slice of life but together, they make up an irresistible pie. Sit back, grab a cup of coffee and enjoy some slices of life because, before you know it, you will have finished the whole thing.
Author: Mark Wilkins ISBN-10: 1936462451   **ISBN-13:** 978-1936462452

Public School Confessions: Stories From The Front Lines of Public Education   SP Loveforce Duo

Teachers, students and administrators come to life and often clash in dozens of stories from the front lines of public education. Within these pages you will meet people who are smart, rebellious and over caffeinated. Some stories will make you laugh, some will make you cry but they will also entertain you and make you think. **Author: Mark Wilkins ISBN-10: 1936462052 ISBN-13: 978-1936462056**

The Faith Trilogy   SP   Loveforce Trio

This Faith Trilogy Paperback includes three faith filled books: What Faith Has Taught Me, The Best Quotes About God and Inspiration for All: Selected Inspirational Writings. **Author: Mark Wilkins ISBN-10**: 1936462516 **ISBN-13**: 978-1936462513

Black in America

Black in America is an exploration of racism in America through essays and poems. It spans from the beginnings of the civil rights movement through today, It includes powerful new poems "Why We Say Black Lives Matter", "Baltimore", "Requiem for Laquan" It takes a look at people who have been lightning rods for race relations in America and has some surprising insights into the people and events that have shaped race relations in America for the past 60 years. It is a powerful work that teaches as it entertains and allows the reader gain new insights. **Author: Mark Wilkins ISBN-10:** 1936462028 **ISBN-13:** 978-1936462025

Controversies

What do Caitlyn Jenner, Donald Trump, Hollywood Sex Scandals, a cure for AIDS, Chinese hackers, Adolf Hitler and Global Warming have in common? They are all at the heart of a controversy and there are stories about them in this unique book that turns tabloid headlines inside out. **Author: Mark Wilkins ISBN-10:** 1936462486 **ISBN-13:** 978-1936462483

Fun for Kidz

This book is the paperback version of School Kidz volumes 1 & 2 and Classic Children's Stories You've Likely Never Heard Before. **Author: Mark Wilkins. ISBN: 978-1936462483**.

www.ingramcontent.com/pod-product-compliance
Lightning Source LLC
Chambersburg PA
CBHW050128280326
41933CB00010B/1290